The Aging Gracefully Pathway: A Toolkit for the Journey is written for the baby boomer market (and, of course, anyone interested in aging with grace and good health). A world-renowned periodontist, the author has used her training in health sciences and medicine while sifting through authoritative information from the last ten to twelve years, to share it with those wanting to age with grace, agility, and good mental and physical health. How many of us know that sugar and refined foods may contribute to Alzheimer's disease? That AGEs (advanced glycation end-products) cause most degenerative diseases and wrinkles? That antioxidants from diet play a leading role in preventing age-related diseases?

Sting said: "I want to get old gracefully. I want to have good posture, I want to be healthy and be an example to my children." At one hundred, Eubie Blake said: "If I'd known I was going to live this long, I'd have taken better care of myself." *The Aging Gracefully Pathway: A Toolkit for the Journey* contains quotes like these plus specific advice for longevity with quality of life, covering everything from the heart to how our skin looks to our posture, brain function, and turning back the internal clock. The entire book is enriched with quotes and easy-to-digest tidbits on how to have a healthy, happy aging experience. A few examples: Cinnamon reduces blood sugar levels, reduces AGEs, is antibacterial and antifungal, and the scent enhances cognitive processing, including attention, memory, and visual-motor speed; the spice turmeric has anticancer and anti-Alzheimer's properties (both from *Ageless Face, Ageless Mind*[21]); "Training on an empty stomach turns on some interesting genetic machinery that is important not only in fat loss but also longevity" (*The Paleo Solution*[15]).

The author's criteria for the selected expert advice were documented consensus, that the ideas made biologic sense, and that they were practical; i.e., they had the quality of everyday usefulness. Individual readers will be able to choose from a plethora of tools, finding what best suits them and their lifestyles. *The Aging Gracefully Pathway: A Toolkit for the Journey* stretches the minds of its readers in a positive way, allowing them to see and take a clear path toward aging gracefully. One of the experts quoted said, "Certainly there will be many paths to successful aging; and there will never be a right way to grow old" (*Aging Well: Surprising Guideposts to a Happier Life*[86]). Compact and easy to read, *The Aging Gracefully Pathway: A Toolkit for the Journey* casts light on many of them.

Oct. 2014

Derek –

THE
AGING
GRACEFULLY
PATHWAY

A Toolkit for the Journey

Here's to a wonderful, graceful aging pathway! :) Cheryl

DR. CHERYL TOWNSEND WINTER

THE AGING GRACEFULLY PATHWAY:
A Toolkit for the Journey

Anti-aging research is here to stay and is
coming of age (so to speak).
(The Aging Myth: Unlocking the Mysteries
of Looking and Feeling Younger[34])

I intend to live forever,
or die trying!

—Groucho Marx

Goal? Die young as
late as possible.
(The Aging Myth[34])

Aging seems to be
the only available way
to live a long time.
—Daniel Francois Esprit Auber

ISBN: 1494876787
ISBN 13: 9781494876784
Library of Congress Control Number: 2014900143
CreateSpace Independent Publishing Platform
North Charleston, South Carolina

DEDICATION:

I dedicate this book to my husband, Morris, for his solid support and input as I wrote this book, to my sister Janice and my favorite (and only) brother, Bill, who are growing older with me, to my departed sisters Anita Louise (Beet) and baby sister Victoria, whose spirits live on in my heart and to all of my nieces and nephews because I want graceful aging for all of them.

ACKNOWLEDGEMENTS:

I want to acknowledge editor, essayist, poet and teacher Sheila Bender for her invaluable help and encouragement to move forward with this book. I would also like to thank Dr. David McKenna for his input about my voice and my sister, Janice, for the time she took to review the book and give me feedback as a potential consumer.

TESTIMONIALS:

Your book sounds like a great project! Very interesting and a lot of valuable information!

How exciting and what a great concept!!

It would be great to get a copy of your book - is it available in print?

That is so amazing! I love that woman. She was my perio Dr until she retired!

Wow you are incredible Cheryl. I'm getting older by the minute and any information would be helpful.

I love what you are doing and would be most happy to feature you!

Your book sounds terrific. I cannot wait to read it.

TABLE OF CONTENTS

PROLOGUE

*There is a fountain of youth: it is your
mind, your talents, the creativity you bring
to your life and the lives of people you
love. When you learn to tap this source,
you will truly have defeated age.*

—Sophia Loren

Twenty-plus years ago, I was among a thousand people in a
ballroom in Bellevue, Washington, only a short distance from
my periodontal practice, listening to an expert panel on aging.
One woman physician, among the seven or so aging special-
ists, quickly captured my attention when she said that the baby
boomers (of which I am one) would change the face of aging.

She said that a number of them would live to be over one hundred; that they would never really retire, but when they stopped working they would find other things, like volunteer or community work or new career directions, to keep them busy; that they would want to leave a legacy; and that they would be healthier and would age more gracefully than any prior generation.

Things that I heard from my boomer patients echoed the aging expert. They were determined to be healthy, and keep their teeth for their lifetime as part of that plan. I also noticed that, like myself, they tended to question things and not just accept them, including being very skeptical of traditional treatment options. They wanted to play an active role in their treatment. It made sense to me that they would question traditional aging and would change the face of it as they became the ageds in our society. As my periodontal practice went on in years, I would also hear my boomer patients echo the aging expert that they wanted their lives to have made a difference, leaving something positive behind when they left the planet.

I definitely fit the profile that the expert on aging painted. I related to everything she said. Since my twenties I had seen myself as living to be over one hundred. I had been exercising regularly since my early thirties and I was fairly health conscious, having regular physicals with my internist from my midthirties on. I had worked on my legacy as a periodontist. I had not seen myself ever truly retiring because I simply had way too much energy for a rocking chair on the porch after life as a gum surgeon. So, the aging expert's predictions really rang true for me. They never left my mind during the twenty-plus years since, as I continued my chosen profession, and now, since my retirement, they ring true even louder than before. What she said had a lot of lasting power for me. I have decided that I want to age as gracefully as I can. I am very conscious of my own aging journey and I want to actively participate in the direction my aging pathway takes. I want to be healthy and I want to make a positive difference in the world before I depart. I embrace that I have the personal power to make all these things happen.

Yes, indeed, boomer I am, I am, and I can relate to this statement from *Juicy Living, Juicy Aging*:[50] "These folks [we baby boomers] have never done anything in a passive way, and they aren't going to take aging lying down." No sir. Not us. We will fight it *tooth* and nail! Aging is a battle we boomers want to win and we believe we can. The dogma that we will age as our parents did does not work for us. All we need are the right tools.

Leading the Anti-Aging Battle Cry!

*Generations before them [baby boomers]
may have faced their senior years with
apprehension, but not so for those trail-
blazers waiting to join the senior ranks.
They've changed everything else about
our world. Now they have the opportunity
to change the face of aging.*

(website article[11])

Interestingly, as my patients and I started to grow old together, I began to notice that some patients aged physically and mentally a lot more gracefully than others. I wondered why, asking myself what were they eating, or drinking, or doing that was making the difference. Or was it all in their genetics? Did they inherit their aging pathway, or did they know something that others did not? Or were they just lucky? Was how the body aged something we could influence? When I would ask some of them what they thought about it, their "genes" was the most common answer, and it was an easy one to accept since we had been taught that this was true. Others had no idea what influenced the way they were aging. The older I became, I began to wonder about how important genetics actually was, and the closer I got to the big fifty, the more curious I got!

Curiosity has always been a big part of who I am. I am curious about pretty much everything in the world around me (well, except maybe stockbroking, which I just find hard to get interested in). As I was exposed to the general requirements of arts and sciences in early college, I began to focus my curiosity on health and well-being, dating back to my first biology course and perpetuated by my dental school education in the late '70s. This curiosity, and the learning that followed, led to a remarkable respect for the human machine. I especially loved and was awed by the physiology of the body.

As I matured in my profession as a gum surgeon, I was also very impressed by and developed respect for how well the body can heal, and the very positive differences in healing that occurred for patients who took care of their gums versus those who did not do their part. It seemed clear to me that, at least for gum tissue, the individual patient played a huge role in how the periodontal treatment turned out. Personal effort making a big difference certainly made sense when I thought about fitness—how fit we are is about how much effort we put in. Maybe the key to aging gracefully wasn't about genetics; maybe aging was about our personal efforts to grow old in a more graceful, healthy way...

In the summer of 2011, I turned sixty, sold my periodontal practice of almost thirty years, and suddenly found myself unemployed for the first time since high school. Each of these major events gave me pause. Together, the remembered words of the expert, my innate curiosity and respect for the human body's potential, the transition in my life to retirement from clinical practice, and reading the book *5: Where Will You Be Five Years From Today?* by Compendium Inc., contributed to my desire and drive to write *The Aging Gracefully Pathway: A Toolkit for the Journey.* I wanted to learn everything I could about aging gracefully, and I wanted to share that knowledge with anyone and everyone who was interested.

AGING GOES BOOM

Statistically, there is no doubt that baby boomers are changing the face of aging. That group of seventy-six million is revolutionizing healthy aging with $3.2 trillion in spending power, according to the Natural Marketing Institute's Healthy Aging/Boomer Database (website article[1]). This same database substantiates that the boomers want to remain relevant and defy "getting older," and that the top drivers of a healthy lifestyle center around weight loss, prevention of disease, and, of course, appearance. The 1990 book *The Age Wave,*[96] states: "The boomers redefine whatever stage of life they inhabit. They have, in fact, already begun to rebuild the later years of life in their own, more youthful image." It calls the boomers true social pioneers, charting the uncertain territory of long life, and author Ken Dychtwald coins the term "age wave" for the massive demographic shift that they are at the center of.

Our timing is excellent. From my review of the literature on aging, I can tell the reader confidently that science has empowered us to do something about aging, providing the tools we need and want. Industry has been paying attention as well, adding their tools into the aging market. Aging product sales— boomers will drive sales from around eighty billion in 2011 to more than 114 billion by 2015 (website article [2])—and the number of plastic surgery procedures (the number of boomers doing cosmetic surgery) is on the rise, according to BabyBoomers.com., (website article [3]) to name two, have supported the idea that we are taking advantage!

Not surprisingly, being as antiestablishment as they have always been, it is also clear that the boomers think about aging differently than their parents. As noted in *Stealing Time*,[40] there is a new paradigm of aging—the belief that aging is a downhill journey is being challenged. The National Institute on Aging reports that body change over time does not inevitably lead to disease (website articles[12]) It is clear to me, after the research for this book, that aging *can* be influenced in a very positive way, creating the opportunity for us to do so. And, there is evidence that we are in fact doing so, including that in the last two decades, the rate of disability among older people has declined dramatically (website article[64]). This is **awesome**! Let's lead the way to more graceful aging, boomers!

For certain, too, we are living longer. "Consistent with the upward trend in longevity, increasing numbers of people are living to be one hundred years old" (*Stealing Time*[40]). As noted in *Living to 100*,[79] which is based on a New England centenarian study, once a rarity, centenarians are the world's fastest-growing age group. There are more than three times as many as there were in 1980, and they are setting the gold standard for healthy aging. In 2009, the UN reported that in the richer countries of the world, life expectancy was lengthening five hours or more every day (*The Aging Myth*[34]). This is around 150 hours each month, and a whopping 1,825 hours (or seventy-six days) each year! At that rate, in less than five years, a full year will be added to our life expectancy.

> Do not regret growing older. It is a
> privilege denied to many.
>
> —Anonymous

A good follow-up question here is: How long is the body designed to last? *The Metabolic Plan*[78] tells us that research shows that the human body has the ability to last about 120 years. This number is our actual life potential or achievable lifetime. YES! But, to live that long with grace, agility, and good mental and physical health will be challenging. We will need some aging tips and tidbits to help us on that journey. Some experts on aging who have studied centenarians have noted that *the key to* preserving *health and vitality lies not in learning how people stay young, but in understanding how they age well* (*Living to 100*[79]). That is what this book is for. I believe I can contribute to both boomers and non-boomers alike helping themselves to age gracefully and with good health by presenting the results of my sifting through the authoritative evidence that is out there on aging—to help us preserve our independence and quality of life for as long as possible.

> We only get one soma [the physical body] in this life, so you have to take care of it if you want it to last.
>
> (*Time of Our Lives*[92])

I have validated that using the tips and tidbits works by using them on, and applying them to, myself as a test-case guinea pig. My most recent RealAge score, from the RealAge Test on their website (website link[3]) is only 54.7 years—a reversal of just shy of eight years compared to my actual birth year age of sixty-two and a half plus. There is also a test available on the web about how long we might live. The Living to 100 Life Expectancy Calculator said my calculated life expectancy is one hundred, but I could live to 103 (website link[17]). My goal is to achieve and maintain that real age reversal, and even subtract a few more years to get an even lower biologic age if I can. In fact, I will take as many years off the actual number as possible so that I can stack them on at the end, taking my one hundred age goal and adding, say, ten to twenty years! I will talk more about RealAge later in the book.

I need to be honest here: I do bring some biases and dogma with me as I write this book. You will notice that there are more references in this book to teeth and gum disease than in most (maybe all) books on aging. This is a big part of who I am (or was, anyway), and it clearly permeates my thinking and my writing. I didn't call myself "gum doctor" all those years for no reason. From age thirty to age sixty, I lived my professional life in the health-care arena, diagnosing and treating gum disease, plus writing and publishing in the scientific literature in conjunction with lecturing all over the country about treating gum disease and, since the late '80s, about how to make someone's smile look prettier.

I took great pride in being part of a patient's health-care team, and the results of our work were very satisfying. Periodontal work is a very focused, albeit narrow, representation of prevention and treatment of disease, coupled with cosmetic procedures that improve smiles (more on smiles in chapter 1, section 2). This too serves as part of my basis for, and interest in, this book.

Another bias that you should know about up front is that on a personal level, I believe in taking only the bare necessity of medications or supplements for the health and well-being issues we face in the aging process. We take too many man-made chemicals in my opinion, and I believe we would be a lot better off if we took more personal responsibility for overcoming as many of our health issues as we can with alternatives like diet and exercise (more on this throughout the book). My clinical practice experience verified this concept, as most patients were successful long term with preventive care and basic, nonsurgical periodontal therapies and their work at home taking care of their teeth and gums, without medications.

Personally, I also had this attitude forced on me to some degree because I am allergic to several medications and sensitive to others. This, coupled with my "minimal medications" view, has always caused second thoughts on anything prescribed for me or recommended off the shelf, or that I might prescribe for my patients. An example of this for me happened about three years ago, when my internist wanted me to take blood pressure medication because I had borderline high blood pressure (HBP). I tried them for a few days, but I didn't like how they made me feel, so, being the boomer that I am, I stopped taking the pills and called my doctor to tell him that I had decided, "No, I am going to get healthier the natural way rather than take those pills." Via lifestyle changes such as additional exercise and improved eating habits, and with help from my research on aging for this book, I did, and I am prescription-free to this day, with my common resting blood pressure being 124/76! Don't get me wrong; sometimes medications are absolutely necessary, and certainly life-saving in many situations, but my thinking is to minimize meds whenever we can by using lifestyle changes as much and as often as possible instead, because I feel the balance has tipped too far in the direction of taking a pill to fix what ails us.

I also firmly believe in preventive and nonsurgical procedures as the first line of treatment, whenever possible. I learned early on in practice that surgery to treat gum disease worked much better and the results lasted much longer when I helped the patient get his/her gums healthy over one to two years with nonsurgical treatment before considering surgical treatment to reshape the gum and bone deformities caused by his/her gum disease. More importantly, besides improved postsurgical results, sometimes getting the patient healthy first eliminated the *need* for gum surgery. This was a stunning and forever professionally altering revelation for me. The plastic surgeon I will talk about at the beginning of chapter 1 had this same philosophy toward facial skin, and twelve years plus down the road, I have yet to have any cosmetic surgery. Not that I won't ever, but so far, so good. There will be more on that story to come.

This preventive, nonsurgical philosophy might also apply to changing the patient's lifestyle to reduce fat before undergoing cosmetic surgery to remove fat without that lifestyle change. (If we have extra fat, should we have someone surgically remove it, or should we figure out how to change our lifestyle, if we can, to permanently remove it without the knife, or at least keep it off after the knife?) Another personal example of this would be that I have been using a healthy diet to keep my weight down and exercise to build muscle tone and ligament strength before going to see an orthopedic surgeon about some proposed knee surgery for torn cartilage.

More than two years has elapsed and I have been able to completely regain all the function in my knee, the swelling is gone, and I have very little pain. I have not yet needed to go see the surgeon, and based on my results so far, I am confident now that I will not need surgery on my knee anytime soon, if ever, even though I have reinjured it a couple of times (including recently twisting my ankle, which twisted my knee). I have been able to rehabilitate it myself each time with very simple at-home exercises, with a small pillow under my knee as I push down toward the floor thirty to thirty-five times for each knee. That's the only special thing I do for my knee but I do it two to three days each week, and I am thrilled with how well I have been able to reduce my pain and restore function with such simple effort. I got excited recently when a local TV station aired a report about a study that showed physical therapy can be as good for a common injury and at far lower costs and less risk than surgery. Loving it!

Again from my experience treating gum disease, and subsequently by doing the research for this book, I developed another bias: I became convinced that our tissues (gum tissue and the rest of our bodies) have more healing potential than we realize. As an aside, did you know that gum tissue has the fastest cell-healing rate in the body? This is important to the body because gum tissue seals our internal body from the external world. Did you also know that gum tissue does not scar, no matter how many times it has been surgically altered? We don't in fact know why, but my long-standing personal theory is the constant moisturizing effects of saliva make a difference. Perhaps this tells us something about skin and postsurgical scarring? Is this food for further thought?

But back to the idea of healing potential—Dr. Joseph Chang said in *The Aging Myth*,[34] "If we give them a chance, our bodies are remarkably intuitive, capable at a cellular level of repairing themselves." This is a powerful observation and it makes perfect biologic sense to me. The design of our vessels is exquisite and sophisticated. It is built to last (120 years, or so it seems). Within that design, I believe, are all the somatic ingredients needed to age gracefully, including healing potential. We can capitalize on that by understanding how it works, accompanied by eating well, exercising, dealing with stress, and all the other aging gracefully ideas that we are going to look at in this book.

As another aside, I was in a conversation with several of my colleagues not too long ago and I asked the group what the maximum age the body was designed for, and a good friend answered 120 years. I asked, "How did you know that?" He replied, "That's what the Bible says." With Google's help I found this: Genesis 6:3: "And the LORD said, My spirit shall not always strive with man, for that he also is flesh: yet his days shall be a hundred and twenty years." Although I don't know exactly how to interpret this, it is interesting to me that this thought goes back that far...

One last bias: educated as a scientist, I tend to discount things that do not make biologic sense to me, so what is in this book has been sifted through my filter of things striking a "chord" with me. In dentistry, having a crown or bridge made on teeth with active gum disease doesn't make biologic sense. You have to get the foundation healthy before you build the superstructure. Other things that make biologic sense to me are things like eating natural foods versus processed foods, dealing with our stress versus taking sedatives to tone down and tune out the stress, and getting the supplements we need from what we eat versus from a bottle, to name only a few. Something that doesn't make biologic sense to me personally would be Botox injections in the arena of cosmetic procedures. Using a poison to completely stop some of our facial expressions is, to me, "contrary" biology. Other examples would be "fillers" in the face, or relying on pills to lose weight without exercising, or not losing the extra pounds before knee or hip replacement surgery, knowing the stress extra weight places on those joints.

The purpose of this book is to sort through and sift out some of what's written about aging, and to try to pull out the "functional/practical" biologically sound ideas that we can use on a daily basis to age gracefully. Along with what makes biologic sense and is practical, a goal in writing this book was to provide us all with tips that had consensus across several experts, sharing their thoughts on various subjects. There's a lot out there! If you use Amazon.com, there are over five hundred thousand titles in the "Health, Mind and Body" section, with more than ninety thousand if you narrow the search to "Personal Health," and still over thirty thousand if you narrow the search further to "Aging." I found my first group of books to review with this method, then I used the subject "Aging" search feature for books from my local library for the remainder of the books I reviewed, along with a few personal recommendations from others along the way.

I came into the research phase of this book prepared, as I could rely on my extensive literature review experience from graduate school, reviewing first titles and book descriptions, then the tables of contents, followed by beginnings and ends of chapters, and then ultimately sifting through the book content from cover to cover. All told, I reviewed 108 books, along with sixty-plus website articles. As a disclaimer, I pulled what "jumped out" at me through my personal lens, which, as I have already pointed out, has some innate bias.

Please note that the expert advice on aging in this book sometimes overlaps or is voiced very similarly by different authorities, but this lends credence to that information because, as I see it, when conclusions are in actuality true, multiple minds from multiple disciplines arrive at them from varying vantage points. When they are not truisms, there tends to be disagreement and multiple opinions on the right answer. More than one purported "right" answer on anything gives me pause, with reason to believe that perhaps the definitive answer is not yet known. In addition, some of the aging "tidbits" may be in more than one section because they apply to more than one aspect of aging.

I am hopeful that providing the volume of quotes and easy-to-digest aging morsels that follow will help us all combat the "if all you have is a hammer, everything looks like a nail" approach to the subject. There are many tools to choose from in our "aging gracefully toolbox"—I want to uncover a big mass of them for the readers' review, letting them pick and choose as they see fit. I firmly believe that we each must create our own path in our own unique way during our lifetimes, and this definitely applies to the aging pathway. As *Aging Well: Surprising Guideposts to a Happier Life*[86] said:

> Certainly there will be many paths to successful aging; and there will never be a right way to grow old.

You will also see throughout this book that I often evaluate choices on aging gracefully from a business perspective: return on investment (ROI). A mentor of mine from graduate school days, Dr. Saul Schluger, first taught me this concept, talking about periodontal therapy decisions. He said each choice has a price. What you have to decide is, is the price worth the outcome. If it is, go for it. If it is not, look for an alternative. This does in fact apply to decisions about periodontal therapy treatment planning, but I believe it applies to much, much more, like maybe *all* our life choices. This is how I try to think about choices I am making. Perhaps the reader may consider this as well.

A list of Internet website addresses that I think may be of interest for additional information and a table of authorities (which is the complete reference list of the books and website articles that I excerpted after review) constitute the end of the book. I encourage the reader to further explore the websites and books as his/her interest determines.

Appropriate here is one of my favorite quotes:

> The truth is rarely pure, and never simple.
>
> —Oscar Wilde

This is one of my credos, my statement of principle/belief professed here formally, and it is true for the information in this book about aging well. I have included what I see as the highlights of *some* of what's out there, considering the widely published broad subject matter and the reach of the Internet. I definitely am not saying that it is all-inclusive, or that it is cut-and-dried, black-and-white, or absolute. Like the information out there about treating gum disease, there are many shades of gray, many still unanswered questions, and of course the individual aging process and individual response to the tools we have available currently, not to mention some disagreement among the authorities.

Periodontics is still an art that is based on science. Aging gracefully is as well. The science is significantly more solid in today's world, but the application of the science is still an art, and must still be customized to the individual to meet his/her needs. Another important caveat to consider is that we do not have to follow every recommendation or suggestion 100 percent of the time. For example, the author of *The Paleo Solution*[15] states that following the Paleo diet 80 percent of the time produces 95 percent of the benefits. We're not perfect out here, as we are ultimately still imperfectly human, and if it is TOO hard, we won't do it! Success comes when we are able to easily incorporate the tips and tidbits into our daily lives. I like to see these small pieces of information on aging gracefully in the light of one of the aging experts, I reviewed: they create a "sparkling" moment; i.e., a challenge to be viewed as an opportunity to change, experiment, push yourself, grow, learn new skills (*Fortytude*[17]).

Having perspective on how hard it is to age is also important. When discussing how tough it is, a former patient said to me: "Getting old is not for wusses." This is oh so very true. I understand it better and better as I age. It takes courage to stay on this planet more than a few decades, and all who read this book and either have a few years already stacked up, or plan a long life, should pat themselves on the back for not only being willing to work at achieving more years, but for trying to do it as gracefully as humanly possible. Here's to you! With attention to aging gracefully, I do believe we can get to the finish line having lived many more years, much more vibrantly. When I am ready to depart this planet, no matter if I am seventy, eighty, ninety, one hundred, or maybe a hundred and twenty, I want to: **skid in sideways...used up, totally worn out, and screaming, "Woo-hoo, what a ride!"** Even though it is somewhat at odds with that statement, I also want my biologic real age to be at *least* ten years younger all the way to the end. But then, I am a boomer. Maybe, after this book, the reader will feel that way, too.

PART 1:

THE OUTSIDE STORY

CHAPTER 1:

OUR BODY AND OUR FIRST IMPRESSIONS

SECTION 1: MIRROR IMAGE: DO YOU SEE WHAT I SEE?

No matter how old you are, you're younger than you'll ever be again.

—Anonymous

INTRODUCTION

"Genes constitute about 1/3 of the factors leading to long life." This was Howard Friedman, quoted in an interview for a

2011 *New York Times* book review (website article[47]) for his and Leslie Martin's book *The Longevity Project*.[12] I was not expecting this. Perhaps it surprises you as much as it did me. This rebukes the long-held myth that we can forecast how we will age based on observing our parents and grandparents, and *throws* out the window the rationale that there is nothing we personally can do to change our aging pathway. We cannot run or hide from aging, but we can definitely impact how our aging pathway unfolds. The million-dollar question, then, is: What constitutes the other two-thirds; i.e., those parts of the aging process that can be altered to improve the long-term outlook? Show us the answers!

Serious, debilitating, or even fatal disease outcomes are potential consequences of aging in an unhealthy, uninformed manner. The loss of independence is another serious possible outcome for us ageds, as are problems with cognition such as dementia and Alzheimer's. I have some very good news to share: *based on what I have learned in writing this book, I can truthfully say that there are tips and tools to help us avoid/reduce these unwanted outcomes*. Knowledge is power, and knowledge about aging is power to fight and swing those nongenetics two-thirds in our favor, changing our aging pathway. This knowledge will hopefully stretch the mind of the reader (as it has stretched the mind of the writer) in a positive way, allowing us all to see and take our clear path toward aging gracefully.

For example, how many of us know that sugar and refined foods may contribute to Alzheimer's disease; that AGEs (advanced glycation end-products from too much sugar) cause most degenerative diseases and wrinkles; that antioxidants from diet play a leading role in preventing age-related diseases? This book will share bits of authoritative information on aging that explores those morsels, along with many more. It provides hundreds of "aging tidbits" for those wanting to age with grace, agility, and good mental and physical health for as long as we are on this planet. Readers will be able to choose from a plethora of tools, finding what best suits them and their lifestyles. The book is enriched with quotes and formatted to make it easy to digest the information.

Choosing to include bits of expert advice on aging was based on them making biologic sense (i.e., being compatible with our bodies and body functions) and having everyday usefulness (i.e., they were practical). It was also important that the tips were easy to incorporate into our lifestyles, without any significant financial or other costs, so that everyone who wants to can choose to age as gracefully as he/she can. For example, did you know the following?

- Cinnamon reduces blood sugar levels, reduces the AGEs (noted two paragraphs back), is antibacterial and antifungal, and the scent enhances cognitive processing, including attention, memory, and visual-motor speed.

- Training on an empty stomach turns on some interesting genetic machinery that is important not only in fat loss but also longevity.

- The spice turmeric has anticancer and anti-Alzheimer's properties.

But before we jump further into the details of aging well, let me tell you the story of how I was first introduced to the idea that I needed to do something about my aging pathway. It was my personal awakening to more graceful aging. Truly amazing how an impending certain decade birthday, a good mirror, and some good light can get our attention. I got very motivated about my pathway to aging gracefully a few months shy of my **BIG** fiftieth birthday. I looked closely in the mirror one day and was horrified by some very baggy eyelid skin, clear wrinkled reflections of my facial expressions, and a very red neck that I didn't want to have when the birthday party came around four months later. As I thought about it, I recalled a lecture on aging from twenty-plus years ago where an aging expert shared the idea that boomers would age more gracefully than any prior generation, and I decided it was time for me to get to it.

I went to a renowned plastic surgeon specializing in eye therapies, whose work I had seen in the process of a trial program; a few local periodontists who did cosmetic "smile" surgery were collaborating with plastic surgeons in our area, and I happened to be one of them. I knew his work was phenomenal because I had seen before-and-after treatment photos of some of his cases. This eye surgery specialist told me that some form of plastic surgery might be useful down the road, but first I needed to see an aesthetician to get my face and neck in better shape before he would even consider surgical treatment. This mirrored my philosophy about treating patients with gum disease and getting them healthy before even considering surgical gum treatment (as I mentioned in the prologue), so I was immediately in sync with the concept and chomping at the bit to go. He referred me to an aesthetician he worked with.

At that time, I didn't have a clue what an aesthetician was, but I took the name and called to set up an appointment. I went to see her as soon as I could. She took special photos and showed me my aging skin. It was shocking to me how much sun damage there was, as I had never been much of a sun worshiper. I was soon to find out that even living in the Northwest, with lots of cloudy or rainy days, sun block is essential on the face to prevent sun-damaged aging. The photos that revealed my damaged skin scared me so much I haven't missed a day of sun protection factor (SPF) 36 cream since! But, it wasn't all bad news, as she shared with me that those of northern European heritage with fair, thin skin like mine tended to respond to the various skin therapies very well. Thank goodness for some ray of hope!

The real shocker came when I asked about the redness on my neck. She said to me: "You have red neck syndrome" (which is the literal sun-damaged skin on the front of the neck). Being a fairly liberal child of the '60s, this really upset me! How could this be? But as they say, it was what it was, and clearly, I had red sun-damaged skin on my neck. It made me think twice before using the term "redneck" after that, not to mention thinking twice before lying in the sun on the beach even on an infrequent occasion! We talked about microdermabrasion and chemical peels. We talked about antioxidants to fight free radicals and retinol-based exfoliation (removing dead skin from the skin's outer layers). This was foreign language to me, as I was completely unaware of any of it. My head was spinning, and all I could think about was, how soon could we start, and how quickly could we reverse my years of bad habits?

She and I went to work right then and there on fixing me up. She helped me learn how to cleanse my skin well, how to moisturize and hydrate, how to use daily sun block (no matter rain or shine), and how retinoids renew skin and vitamins C and E (antioxidants) protect it from sun damage and harmful free radicals. I also learned about mineral-based cosmetics, and I became personally very familiar with microdermabrasion, a number of chemical peel treatments, and several masks, along with other skin therapies. I found the whole process to be very appealing and relaxing, with wonderful smells and textures to the various skin therapies in conjunction with lots of facial massage while resting comfortably in a heated spa bed listening to soothing music. I also noted, as did others, that I was looking decidedly younger—it was working!

I became a true convert, to the point where starting or ending the day without my daily facial skin regimen didn't feel right, sort of like not being able to start the day without brushing and flossing. More on this later in section 2, and in a couple of other spots—okay, maybe several spots—throughout this book.

I still use this same skin regimen today, more than twelve years later and I still see my aesthetician at the medical skin clinic/spa that I started out at. Over that time, I have only added Clarisonic sonic cleansing and the Opal sonic device (more on these later on). In retrospect, I am certain it would have been better if I had started even younger (it certainly is easier to make changes when we are younger, but I think we benefit no matter our age). But it took that looming fiftieth birthday to really get my attention enough to take a hard look at myself in the mirror, which created the momentum to do something about it—and boy, am I glad I did!

Looking back, I am surprised at myself, because I knew that to keep the mouth healthy and "young," we had to have a super strong commitment to take meticulous care of our teeth and gum tissue. But I had never thought much about our facial skin before I met the aesthetician, even though structurally, gum is the same as the skin on our face. I started flossing my teeth in the early '70s at about age twenty, but it took me until 2001, age fifty, to get the message about caring for my facial skin.

IT'S MORE THAN JUST ABOUT OUR FACE

My research of the aging experts has taught me something that is critical to understand: looking/acting/being more youthful is about a lot more than our skin we see or the wrinkles on our faces. Wrinkles on our faces are just *one* sign that we may not be aging as well as we could. The rest of the external body ages in tandem with the face, as does the internal body. We don't think about that much because it is the face that dominates the impression of age, but poor aging of the skin would foretell poor aging of the rest of our bodies. Actually, now that I am much more knowledgeable about aging, I think most worrisome is not the face, which is what got me started and which we see in the mirror fairly often, but where we don't look, or are unable to look, to evaluate how we are aging.

As the book progresses, we will look at it all, head to toe and inside out, taking a totalitarian point of view. The book is divided into three parts, to share with you information first about the external body, then the internal body, and finally the "spirit" or soul that the body houses. Within these three major divisions, I will share the authoritative details and subtleties about aging and aging well that I have uncovered.

Here is some food for thought before we move on: an authoritative example of "it's more than just about your face" is the following from the book *SuperHealth*.[59] This is the aging expert's list of the possible signs of poor aging (be certain to take note of number two):

Signs of poor aging inside and generating too many free radicals while being short on antioxidants:

1. *Dark circles under the eyes.*
2. *Bleeding gums.*
3. *Poor posture.*
4. *Dull, dry, and wrinkled skin.*

FOUR THINGS TO BEGIN THIS JOURNEY

Of course I'm in shape—
isn't round a shape?

—Anonymous

Okay. We have the foundational concept that we can affect two-thirds of how we age. Now the question we have to answer is how do we begin a pathway to graceful aging? Where is the starting line? How do we figure out what direction to take? What does the finish line look like? I have already introduced this discussion by talking about my own personal interaction with the face in the mirror shortly before the looming fifth-decade birthday. A mirror is critical at the onset of the journey, but as was recently discussed, this pathway of aging is about a lot more than looking at your face in a mirror. That initial step, to evaluate how things look at the starting line, best includes the entire body. I have divided the evaluation into four things that I feel we must do to get started down our aging gracefully pathway.

MIRROR, MIRROR ON THE WALL

The first step, and one of the most essential, is that look in the mirror: it is very important that you take some time to see yourself as if you were an outside observer, asking the question, what do others see when they first see me? How old do I look? While looking intently in that mirror, ask yourself this:

How old would you be if you didn't know how old you are?

—Satchel Paige

We may not like what we see, but by truly "seeing" ourselves and acknowledging what we don't like, only then can we begin the process of making positive changes on the path to the way we want to be, all the while turning back the clock as much as we can.

So, to start our aging gracefully pathway, we must step our body (naked gives the most complete perspective) in front of a full-length mirror and turn right and left a few times, turning our head from side to side to get a 360-degree perspective. Some of us will need to wear our glasses to get a true view of the subject. The first big obstacle to aging as gracefully as we can is us not knowing how our soma (body, distinct from the mind or soul) looks. It may have been awhile (or maybe a very long while) since we looked at our full and complete selves in the mirror, with good lighting and eyewear, as needed. What do others see when they look at us? How does our skin look? Does it have vibrancy? Or does it appear dry and crepe-like? What shape are we in? Is there extra padding in places that the padding isn't very welcome? Is there little "extra" to grab on to anywhere, or is there plenty to hold on to?

Are our shoulders straight up and down, or slumped and rounded? How are those wrinkles we've been cultivating doing? How about our hands? How old do they look? Is there some extra skin under the chin or along the jaw that we wish wouldn't show up in every recent photo? Walking toward the mirror, do we walk with our feet pointing straight forward, or in a more "duck-like" manner? Do we pick up our feet when we walk, or do we shuffle? Are we fluid when we move, or are our movements a little shaky or stiff?

These are some tough questions, and they may be somewhat painful to answer, but they are critical for an honest, thorough assessment, top to bottom and front to back. And don't be shy about looking at yourself this way because this journey requires getting used to it. As we continue down this aging gracefully pathway, it has to be understood that this is not a one-time look. To check on our progress, we must repeat this mirror evaluation frequently. I do this a time or two every month when I change clothes or before I shower, and it isn't always pretty because, like all humans, I am perfectly imperfect.

Perhaps taking all this in at one point in time is too much. If we don't want to look that closely at the whole body in the buff in a mirror with good lighting and our glasses, we can start the journey by going to RealAge.com (website link[3]) and taking their Skin Test, which will give us a ballpark age for our skin after we answer some questions (once we have washed our skin and gotten a good view of our face in the mirror). The age calculated at the end will give us an idea of how our skin appearance age compares with our chronologic age.

I warn you, though, even this one step can be kind of eye-opening! I don't think this method is as powerful as my earlier recommendation, but it certainly gets us thinking about some of the detail signs of aging. To really make this work, however, we will, at some point, still need to take a full-body look in the mirror—with clothes at first, if need be—to evaluate our shape, our posture, how we walk, how our hands look, etc. If it is easier to look in baby steps, that is okay. What's important is the looking and getting used to relooking.

The second step on the journey is to hone in on the component parts of the face that speak so loudly and easily about age.

We can start by smiling at ourselves in the mirror. How does our smile look? Are we "long of tooth"? Or do we have healthy pink gums and tooth lengths that meet our upper lip line when we smile? Next, let's take a look at our hair. What kind of frame is our hair for our face? Does it date us? Does it enhance our face, or draw attention to things we would rather it didn't? Are there opportunities here to knock our appearance age back a few years? Is our skin "tight" or not so much?

The third required step is that we must get on the scale to evaluate where our weight is, relative to the healthy weight for our height. The following is a table from the web to help you with this. Carrying five, ten, fifteen, or thirty or more pounds of extra weight around every day, all day long, is very hard on our bodies; our soma is not designed for weight that exceeds what our frame was engineered for. That extra weight is also very hard on the aging process itself, which we will talk a lot more about in part 2, chapter 2.

Carrying that kind of load can injure our knees, contribute to diseases such as diabetes and heart disease, and can slow us into too much inactivity. The list goes on and on, with the negative outcomes feeding on themselves! I don't like to harp, but looking in a mirror frequently, and weighing ourselves once a week or so, is our feedback for how we are doing on the physical end of the aging process. I even go so far as to sometimes grab the skin on my lower back, or under the back of my upper arms (which my sister, Janice, calls chicken wings), to see how I am doing with the extra padding or flapping skin in those areas.

I also keep my scale close to the shower door, where I see it every day, to remind me to weigh myself once a week or so before I get into the shower. Recently, WebMD reported about this, saying that people who succeed at losing weight and keeping it off weigh themselves often, research shows. A step on the scale at least once a week seems to build awareness best (website article[52]). The more comfortable we are with checking ourselves out and looking at the number on the scale, the better use we can make of all the fabulous information out there about aging gracefully.

	Female Height to Weight Ratio				Male Height to Weight Ratio		
Height	Low	Good	High	Height	Low	Good	High
4' 10"	100	115	131	5' 1"	123	134	145
4' 11"	101	117	134	5' 2"	125	137	148
5' 0"	103	120	137	5' 3"	127	139	151
5' 1"	105	122	140	5' 4"	129	142	155
5' 2"	108	125	144	5' 5"	131	145	159
5' 3"	111	128	148	5' 6"	133	148	163
5' 4"	114	133	152	5" 7"	135	151	167
5' 5"	117	136	156	5' 8"	137	154	171
5' 6"	120	140	160	5' 9"	139	157	175
5' 7"	123	143	164	5' 10"	141	160	179
5' 8"	126	146	167	5' 11"	144	164	183
5' 9"	129	150	170	6' 0"	147	167	187
5' 10"	132	153	173	6' 1"	150	171	192
5' 11"	135	156	176	6' 2"	153	175	197
6' 0"	138	159	179	6' 3"	157	179	202

This is the baseline data. Take note of what you would like to change to improve the overall look of the vessel, to turn the clock back a few years. Try to be very specific with this list. *I am a firm believer that you can't get somewhere unless you know where it is that you are trying to go.* The list of desired improvements becomes our goal list to make our vision of graceful aging a reality. With due consideration for our age, some of us may want to jot the list down on paper. Of course, we can also remind ourselves of the list by checking in the mirror every so often, which allows us to keep our eye on our goals, both literally and figuratively with our mind's eye.

The last, and perpetual, thing we must do for this journey to better aging has already been mentioned. That is, a periodic reevaluation in the mirror is critical to success, because it helps you redefine that goal list and demonstrates your successes, for which you then reward yourself (and it is important to do this in some fashion) to help motivate the continuance of the fight to age well.

Speaking of rewards, the ways to reward ourselves are as plentiful as the individuals interested in aging well. A kind of reward I hadn't thought of is an idea offered on a WebMD slideshow titled *24 Ways to Lose Without Dieting* (website article[28]).

It suggested hanging an old favorite dress, skirt, or that pair of jeans that is only a little too snug (so we can reach the goal in a relatively short time) where we see them every day, to help us "keep our eyes on the prize." Being able to slip into that clothing item without strain is an awesome reward to keep us going, and it makes looking in that mirror much more fun. When we achieve that, we can replace the article of clothing with another "fave" that's a little too small, and so on.

Okay. We have completed the necessary four steps to begin the journey on our aging gracefully pathway. We have collected the baseline data and the initial assessment is finished. As we go forward now, we will look at the specific "tidbits" on aging as well as inspirational quotes. There are many of both of these in this book. The idea is for the individual reader to choose the ones that jump out, that "click" with or resonate with him/her; i.e., that are a good fit. The pathway to aging gracefully is definitely an individual process, and no two of us will do it exactly the same. My hope is that with lots of choices, anyone reading this will be able to put together the toolkit that works for him or her. That is a key point. Said well in *The Everything Anti-Aging Book*:[55] "No single anti-aging regimen works for everyone."

SECTION 2: LET'S FACE IT: OUR SMILE, HAIR, AND SKIN

I want to die young at a ripe old age.

—Ashley Montagu

My journey started with my face. We have already discussed the concept that there is much more to aging than our faces, but let's face it, it does play a huge and initial role in the estimation of how old we are. Of course, the face is a composition of several features, but I have chosen to talk about the three that I feel have the greatest influence: smile, hair, and skin. These components of first impressions provide us a sense of who this person is, what his/her "genre" is, and provokes a reaction from us as to how we might interact with him/her. I think it is safe to say that we all want to make a good first impression, and that if we had a choice, we would choose to look as young as possible for as long as possible—maybe fooling everyone right up to the end, which is my personal goal! So, let's take a closer look at these three major players in the composition of our face.

"LONG OF TOOTH"

Let's start with the smile (imagine that, and don't forget, I warned you about this bias in the prologue). There are a number of ways for us to think about our smile's impact on our aging, and they are in the order of how we will consider them.

- *Smiling can take years off your age.*

- *Taking care of our smile can prevent gum disease and its aging consequences, improving longevity.*

- *How we care for our smile is part of the overall picture of how we care for ourselves in general, speaking volumes about our priorities and values.*

> **Anti-Aging Quick Tip: Did you know that a study showed that facial images that were smiling were age-underestimated by twenty-four months? Curve up those lips and take two right off the top! (*The Latest Science on Aging*[89])**

What a great start! Not only does a smile make us look younger, it also helps us succeed in business, fill our social calendars, and get more romance (website article[35]). But, not all smiles are created equal. Did you know that one of the potential consequences of gum disease is a shrinking of the gums around the teeth, wherein the "long of tooth" reference to being older lies? Another consequence of gum disease is tooth loss. Another? Bad breath. These consequences can really age our smile, and therefore the human that is attached to that smile. The good news is, this can be avoided with proper care, including brushing and flossing *every day*, along with regular checkups and cleanings, and periodontal treatment (remember, being retired, I no longer have a vested interest), if needed.

So, if we want to protect that youthful smile from gum disease, I would ask that we consider this thought: ***brush and floss only the ones you wish to keep, and skip the rest.*** I can't begin to enumerate how many times over these thirty-plus years I have made this statement to friends, family, patients, strangers, whoever would listen—it has been way too many to count. But it's true, and in this case, the truth really **is** simple. The reason to brush and floss is to prevent gum disease. There is often some confusion about decay being the main dental problem, but let me set the record straight. The big dental problem that results in tooth loss in adults is **NOT** decay, but rather gum (or more formally, periodontal) disease. Seventy percent of all adult tooth loss is due to periodontal disease, with it being a disease largely of those over thirty-five. As age increases, the incidence of gum disease increases, and new data shows us that one out of every two Americans over thirty have it!

Here is a perspective you may have never heard or thought of. I used to tell my periodontal patients: if you only have time to use one tooth-cleaning tool, skip brushing and do the flossing. Now, this may be somewhat exaggerated, but the concept is that floss cleans below the gum about three millimeters (the depth of the normal, healthy "mote" between gum and tooth), which has a very powerful effect on preventing/reversing gum disease, and therefore tooth loss. If everyone younger than thirty-five added flossing to the tooth care routine, traditional periodontal therapy would disappear for lack of patients.

If preventing "stinky" gum disease and tooth loss is not enough motivation, take the MouthAge Test on the RealAge. com website (website link[3]). When I took this test recently, my mouth age came out to thirty-nine years—a whopping twenty-three years less than my actual age—so check it out! Think about this—flossing daily can turn back the aging clock for us in a huge way, at very minimal expense, and with merely the level of effort that it takes to become a daily habit, after which doing it will become part of our normal lifestyle routine.

Anti-Aging Quick Tip: Daily flossing can provide immediate benefit in terms of starting on the path to healthy gum tissue, with the long-term benefit of increased longevity and keeping your teeth as long as you want them.

This brush and floss daily thing is not only about protecting a youthful smile. RealAge.com declares: boost longevity in one minute by, yes, you guessed it, flossing. On the same website, an article, titled "How Flossing is Linked to Overall Health", tells readers that neglecting their teeth and gums may even lead to erectile dysfunction, in addition to heart disease and diabetes (website article[45]). Who would have thought? The idea of losing my teeth scared me enough to get me flossing every day since the early '70s, and I simply cannot start my day without thoroughly cleaning all that bacteria off my teeth because it grosses me out! My mouth does not feel right until I brush and floss. But then, some might classify me as a bit, or perhaps more than a bit, anal retentive! Yet, with all the mounting evidence, maybe I was right all these almost forty years about the importance of flossing and gum disease...

> Some of the earliest signs of diabetes, cancer, immune disorders, hormone imbalances and drug issues show up in the gums, teeth and tongue long before a patient knows anything is wrong. And there's growing evidence that oral health problems, particularly gum disease, raise the risk of some illnesses.
>
> (website article[17])

Need more evidence for daily flossing and brushing? A study from Stockholm, Sweden, followed the health of 1,390 people for twenty-four years and found that high levels of dental plaque are linked to the chance of dying from any cause, but particularly cancer, thirteen years earlier than expected (website article[29]). In addition, the Mayo Clinic advises that all of the following physical conditions may be linked to oral and dental health: endocarditis (infection of the inner lining of the heart); cardiovascular (heart) disease; premature birth and low-birth-weight pregnancies; diabetes; HIV/AIDS; osteoporosis; Alzheimer's; other conditions, including immune system disorders, and eating disorders (website article[30]). A study supported by the National Institutes of Health in the journal *Circulation* reported that, "Older adults who have higher proportions of four periodontal-disease-causing bacteria inhabiting their mouths also tend to have thicker carotid arteries, a strong predictor of stroke and heart attack"(website article[61]).

Another study, done by researchers at the University of California, followed 5,500 elderly people for eighteen years and found that those who reported brushing less than once a day were up to 65 percent more likely to develop dementia than those who brushed daily (website article[31]). When I posted this tidbit on LinkedIn, an assistant professor replied that he had carefully reviewed epidemiological evidence about dementia twenty years ago and shared this: "I believe improved dental care is partly responsible for the lower rates of dementia in the current generation of older adults and elders." If that is not enough, a new study finds significant associations between antibodies (our bodies' soldiers that help fight disease) for multiple mouth bacteria and the risk of pancreatic cancer, indicating they too may be related (website article[32]).

Recent information indicates that gum disease may even play a role in arthritis. A website article reported that "Scientists have found traces of gum bacteria in the knees of people with rheumatoid arthritis and osteoarthritis." The study, published in the *Journal of Clinical Rheumatology*, adds more evidence of the link between oral health and poor health in general. The article author states: "Want healthy knees? Then you better floss your teeth" (website article[44]).

> While an old saying advises that "the eyes are the window to the soul," modern dental research says the mouth provides an even better view of the body as a whole.
>
> (website article[17])

Said another way, if the eyes are the window to the soul, the mouth is the window to the body. To summarize, a healthy, aesthetic, and youthful smile is one very good reason to brush and floss. Preventing bad breath is another (active bacterial gum disease does not smell very good, which could interfere with your interpersonal relations). Avoiding the need to see a periodontist is another, not to mention that since gum disease has been shown to have a number of linkages to serious diseases such as diabetes, heart disease, stroke, Alzheimer's, lung disease, various cancers, etc., preventing the disease from starting, or reversing it if already present, may have a major, life-changing effect on your aging process.

Our smile represents us in all we do; it is critical to our well-being. It deserves a high spot on the priorities list. Stated well in website article[6] is this: "Take care of your teeth [and gums, of course] and they will take care of you." So, did I mention my gum bias?

> Letting your eyes, ears, mouth, and teeth fall into disrepair can have far reaching consequences for your general health, especially as you age.
>
> (Healthy Aging for Dummies[81])

As an aside, did you know that eating certain foods can improve your eye health? RealAge.com (website article[37]) lists seven choices: kale, oranges, peanuts, kidney beans, salmon (I feel very lucky that I live in the Northwest!), whole grains, and apricots. Also helpful is eating a wide variety of fruits and vegetables, plus choosing healthy fats and high-fiber carbs, while reducing your intake of red meat, sugars, and refined flours. WebMD adds that foods that are good for your circulation are good for not only your heart but your eyes. Their list includes citrus fruits, dark leafy greens, whole grains, beans, peas, peanuts, oysters, lean red meat, and poultry, along with carrots, and yellow or orange fruits and veggies (website article[49]).

Back on topic, how we care for our smiles, eyes, and ears speaks volumes about how we care for ourselves in general, including personal health, hygiene, and fitness. Can't you hear our mothers' voices here? They believed checking out a potential mate's teeth and gums was an important measure of health and beauty; this also foretold how good a mate these people would be based on how they cared for themselves, and their priorities and values. What they didn't know then is that teeth are also a good indicator of the prospective mate's health and longevity, not to mention procreativity...

FACE FRAME: TAKE TEN (YEARS) OFF YOUR FACE

Hair brings one's self-image into focus; it is vanity's proving ground. Hair is terribly personal, a tangle of mysterious prejudices.

—Shana Alexander

The frame of the face is, of course, another important part of those first impressions we make. There are two aspects to consider when evaluating the role hair plays in aging: there is the aesthetic role of the actual haircut/style and there is what our hair might be telling us about our overall health. An ill-fitting haircut/hairstyle can make us look years, or even many years, older. I see my hairstylist every six to eight weeks and change my hairstyle once or twice a year. Lately I frame my conversations with her around styles that are more current and age-enhancing. If we are looking good, it leads to feeling good. Feeling good leads to a more positive outlook and self-image, and a more positive message to those around us. This is part of rewriting the face of aging. Let's show those who come after us how to do it as well as it can be done! Let's get the most out of every opportunity we have to age gracefully, including our hairstyle! Boomers we are, we are!

So, let's look at our hairdo: Is it a nice frame that highlights our face, or is it a distraction? Would it benefit from a more modern cut versus the one we've had for a while (or a long while)? A little effort in this area makes a huge difference in how we look and feel, and can truly date us if it hasn't changed in a while (or a very long while). Like our smile, hair speaks volumes about attention paid to self, how well we have kept up as time has gone by, what kind of effort we make to look good each day and how much we care about the way we present ourselves to the rest of the world. There's a lot more to our hairstyle than what we may think at first glance.

A simple web search will reveal a number of websites that offer hairstyle ideas that can make us look ten years younger. We can Google hairstyles for older men and women, looking for something that "speaks" to us so that we can print it out to take to our next haircut appointment. A more youthful outcome can happen in merely an hour with simple changes to the style and maybe color of our hair. Face-framing layers can make our face look softer and younger but still allow our eyes to pop. Fine-tuning of our hairstyle can give our skin a lovely glow. In addition, according to some experts, it is not true that you should always go lighter in color as you get older, as some have suggested. It's about what looks and feels good. From *Forever Cool*:[70] "dull and lifeless hair is aging." Why not have it sparkle a little, be a little modern, have a little "spice" to it?

As you age, it also makes sense to re-evaluate your hair, makeup and clothing...There are many wonderful styles that can make you feel current, vital, and somewhat hip.

(Juicy Living, Juicy Aging[50]*)*

As far as hair and health go, like skin, too much sun can damage our hair, turning it into a brittle, dry mop that breaks and splits easily (website article[34]). Crash diets can also damage our hair, because luscious-looking hair does need nutrients and very-low-calorie diets can stunt hair growth or leave it dull and limp. If the nutritional deficiency is big enough, as in eating disorders, hair can actually fall out (website article[34]). There are also foods you can eat for healthy hair, according to RealAge.com in one of their tips: green tea, walnuts, and salmon; brightly colored fruit; beans, whole grains, and other vitamin B-rich foods; dark green veggies, dark sesame seeds; and avocados (website article[26]). WebMD (website article[27]) adds sweet potatoes (which I love), poultry, oysters, eggs, Greek yogurt, and low-fat dairy products to the list.

In addition, from *You Being Beautiful*,[93] by the cofounders of RealAge, comes these tips about caring for you hair: blot your hair with a towel versus rubbing or winding it into a tight turban (hair is most vulnerable when wet); use low heat if you use a dryer; never use ceramic appliances on hair; treat your hair like fine silk—delicately; apply conditioners daily (you don't have to shampoo daily, however); and eat well (as noted earlier). WebMD (website article[4]) gives the following tips for beautiful hair:

Boost thin hair with silicone.
Eat fish and nuts for healthy hair.

Protect shine with lukewarm water.
Mend split ends with conditioners that
have protein.
Use hair product on dry root area first for
volume.
Skip high-powered blow-dryers.
Brush less to limit hair loss.
Avoid styles like tight ponytails or braids
that damage hair.
Use gentle color to cover grays.
Use conditioners to neutralize static.
Use a pick instead of a brush for curly hair.
Avoid extreme color changes.
Protect your hair before styling with
conditioner.
Protect hair from the sun.
Take time out from styling.

SKIN TIGHT?

Looking in a mirror shook my sense of my youthfulness with vivid facial signs of aging. Does it yours? As we discussed at the beginning of section 1, skin, especially facial skin (but also hands, arms, legs), can very quickly and easily convey "older"—or maybe better, "younger." As I talked about early in the book, this is the area that really got me going on my better aging pathway. I spend time every morning and every night (at roughly a 90 percent plus level) working at the skin care regimen I learned about twelve years ago. I am very aware of the effort that is required to keep this going, especially when we are "dog" tired at the end of the day, but it really pays off! It's a choice of making the efforts to reap the rewards versus not bothering or putting it off until tomorrow (which doesn't always work out so well). It is something we can keep close tabs on, too: we can check it out every time we take that look in the mirror.

And we aren't the only ones checking it out—others do so every time they see us face-to-face or computer camera to computer camera. Did you know that skin is our biggest organ? There's a lot of exposure there! So let's start this discussion with some skin basics, here from *1001 Ways to Stay Young Naturally*:[39] Deep breaths, fruits and veggies, hydration, exercise, moisturizer when skin is damp, get essential fats, stop smoking, get sleep, de-stress. Another review of anti-aging skin basics from *The Skin Commandments*[76] that most of the aging experts I reviewed agree with:

The Skin Commandments

1. *Never tan.*
2. *Honor your skin (wear sunscreen no matter rain or shine, cleanse, hydrate, exfoliate plus be gentle with your skin)*
3. *Cleanse correctly; i.e., gentle cleanser with warm water and smooth-textured washcloth or clean hands.*
4. *Hydrate holistically; i.e., apply moisturizer (plumps up fine lines and makes skin look younger) when skin is damp, drink plenty of water and eat lots of raw, water-rich, plant-based foods, plus avoid excess alcohol and caffeine.*
5. *Exfoliate effectively; i.e., nightly with a retinoid-based product, at-home peels one time per week, and use loofah scrubs, shower*

scrunchies and soft-bristled brushes on the body and pumice stones on hands and feet.

6. *Fight free radicals (avoid UV rays, which lead to photoaging, smoking, alcohol in excess, oxidative foods and skin-care products with harmful additives). Use topical antioxidants (vitamins C and E)—second most important to sunscreen.*

Please note that this list also included a couple of things that that I have an innate bias against, so in full disclosure, I left those off.

Beyond those basics, it makes biologic sense to me that our skin would benefit from massage, stimulation, and exercise to keep it younger-looking, much like the rest of our body. For me, a good indicator is that aestheticians do a significant facial massage as part of any facial treatment. Facial massages can relax the muscles and stimulate blood flow and lymph circulation (which helps our body by removing and destroying waste, debris, dead blood cells, pathogens, toxins, and cancer cells). There are many references in the library or on the web about facial massage techniques we can benefit from.

As for exercise and the face, there are two ways to look at it: full body exercise and exercising the facial muscles. *Bill Frank's Forever Young*[45] says: "Your face needs and will respond positively to exercise." I like the way my skin looks after a good workout at the gym, or after yoga class. It has vibrancy and color. You can see the benefits easily in that mirror, mirror on the wall.

Anti-Aging Quick Tip: A trip to the gym is great for the body, but it also looks good on your face.

With regard to specific facial muscle exercising, think about it. We could do these exercises in the car as we drive, in our tub as we bathe, in the comfort of our favorite chair as we watch TV: **no gym required.** Exercising in general is good for our skin tone, and exercising of specific facial muscles may be as well. You may have seen the bumper sticker or T-shirt proclaiming: "Exercise, the Poor Man's Plastic Surgery." I am guessing they were not talking about facial muscle exercise, but it might apply, so give that some thought.

Face It

☐ Facial exercise can keep your face and eyes youthfully energized.

☐ Try fingertip massage, acupuncture, reiki
(Japanese technique for stress reduction and
relaxation), ko bi do (ancient Japanese facial massage for beauty and health); use lip exercises.

(1001 Ways to Stay Young Naturally[39])

But, in my search for tips that aging experts agree on, I
must share this: not all aging experts agree on facial exercise.
Drs. Roizen and Oz, RealAge.com cofounders, believe that exercising facial muscles is "a sure-fire way to increase wrinkles" (*You
Being Beautiful*[93]). I have also seen this opinion on WebMD. This
is one bit of aging information that I am still on the fence about
after my research for this book because, as you may recall, my
philosophy is that if there are differing opinions about a subject,
it usually means that the real answer is still unknown. I include
it here for the reader to consider and for completeness' sake.

I also am a firm believer in getting the right skin products
for your skin type and age, to assist in your skin's "vibrancy"
while enjoying the "massage" benefits of applying them. From
Colour Me Younger,[74] there are some topical agents that I use and

aging experts recommend that are very beneficial: retinoids, which are chemically related to vitamin A, help renew your skin, and vitamins C and E, which are antioxidants, protect skin from damaging free radicals. The use of these agents is supported by many aging authorities. In *You Being Beautiful*,[93] it was noted that vitamins A, C, and E are inactivated by UV light, so they are best used at night.

Here is one of the more interesting morsels on skin anti-aging: you can use olive oil to decrease UVB (sun's shortwave ultraviolet rays that some think are more damaging) damage by massaging it into skin, scalp and hair, nails, and lips.[93] In addition, I have seen a number of web-based ideas about natural oils for skin, including argan (a Moroccan all-star), coconut (Caribbean women swear by it), jojoba (from the seeds of a shrub native to the Sonoran Desert), murala (Kenyan women have used for centuries), pomegranate, avocado, and grape seed oil. I have even seen/heard of using castor oil, or emu oil! Speaking of oils, did you know that catnip essential oil is ten to twenty times more effective than DEET at repelling mosquitoes? (I saw that on a website ad—this is clearly off the track—it must be the cat influence from my five furry, four-legged kids around here.)

Getting back on track, where else might we look to turn the face clock back a few years? Are there newly developed technologies we might use? We have options. This is a good time to be aging, with all that is known and all that is available. A few years back, I read the book *Raving Fans*, and let me tell you for certain, I am a raving fan of two relatively new potential "wonder" ultrasonic products for facial care that have emerged: Clarisonic and Opal, or the "Skin Care Pair."

The Clarisonic is a sonic cleansing tool with study results that showed that after twelve weeks of use, over 80 percent of users perceived improvement in their skin. I have been using it almost five years now, on the original recommendation of one of my hygienists. I don't like to do my face washing anymore without my Clarisonic, as nothing else has ever gotten my face as squeaky-clean. Ultrasonic toothbrushes dramatically improved brushing results and healthier gums, leaving teeth squeaky-clean on brushing surfaces—another overlap between gum tissue and skin!

It also makes biologic sense to me that it improves product absorption, so we get more return on investment (ROI), or "bang" for our buck, and since those products are not in the least cheap, this is very important. The fact that aestheticians in spas, medical skin clinics/spas and beauty centers are also using it as part of their anti-aging treatments is strong validation from the skin experts. These products have been put through vigorous research to ensure that their usefulness is proven via only the best research protocols.

Sonic Cleansing Research

- Removes six times more makeup than manual cleansing.
- Leads to 61 percent greater absorption of vitamin C when compared to manual cleansing.
- Helps improve the appearance of skin tone, texture, elasticity and firmness in mature skin.
- Makes skin look and feel softer, smoother and healthier.
- Is safe and gentle enough to use twice a day.

> (Clarisonic website article[7])

The Opal device is a sonic infusion tool. I use it on fine wrinkles around the eyes, forehead, and upper lip area, although it has only been studied for eye use. I began to see results by the end of the second week, and I use it every day to maintain that improvement. My skin not only looks better, but I think this kind of stimulation is very good for the skin. And it feels oh so good, too!

Sonic Infusion Benefits

- *Immediately hydrates, leaving skin feeling refreshed.*
- *Noticeably firmer skin after four weeks.*
- *Reduces appearance of fine lines and puffiness in as little as eight weeks.*
- *Gentle for daily use.*
- *Can be layered with your own eye cream.*
- *Improves skin texture.*

MORE TIPS AND TRICKS, OR TREATS?

Okay, what other rocks can we turn over to help us improve the look of our skin? There are some additional areas where we might effect change to fight and win the war on aging skin. If we are aware of what causes aging of the skin, we should be able to figure out what to do about it. The big skin-aging culprits that came up often from the aging experts I reviewed were UV rays, environmental toxins like exhaust fumes, pesticides, etc., and the food we eat, sugar being high on the list of bad aging foods.

Sugar is the worst thing for skin.

(The Anti-Aging Solution[41])

Other threats to youthful skin include stress, smoking, alcohol, insufficient sleep, and lack of exercise, as noted in *Ageless Face, Ageless Mind*[21] and in agreement with many other aging authorities.

> ## Anti-Aging Quick Tip: Avoid sugar and fight off a major aging enemy!

By avoiding sugar and the other threats to our skin, we can fight two of the three major skin-aging enemies: free radicals from oxidation and advanced glycation end-products (AGEs). We will talk in more detail about free radicals and AGEs in part 2, chapter 2, and diet much more extensively in chapter 3. Since facial wrinkles are such a big part of any discussion about aging, I want to mention here, though, that besides sugar, there are certain foods that are classified specifically as "wrinkle protectors" and certain ones that are "wrinkle promoters." For you to "digest" is this list from *Your Skin, Younger*[69] of protectors (note how similar they are to the list for healthy hair):

Food Wrinkle Protectors: Omega-3 fish. Veggies, especially dark green. Whole-grain cereals. Eggs. Olive oil. Nuts and legumes. Low-fat diary. Tea and water. Dark colored fruits. Zinc in fish and seafood. Ginger and turmeric should be top choices for youthful skin.

(Your Skin, Younger[69])

Important: turmeric has really been a "standout" for anti-aging in my research. It has been described as a spice for the ageless. It slows the process of aging and promotes youthfulness in all organ systems, including skin (*Ageless Face, Ageless Mind*[21]), among other anti-aging qualities, which we will talk more about in chapter 3, section 3. I try to use a little turmeric several times each week now that I know its high value in the fight against aging. Now, consider the promoter list:

Food Wrinkle Promoters: Processed meats. High-fat dairy. White potatoes. Butter and overall saturated fat. Margarine. Baked goods. Soft drinks.

(Your Skin, Younger[69])

Of course, there are also professional options that offer anti-aging advice and assistance for more youthful skin. The armamentarium offered by the teams of aestheticians, physician assistants, and plastic surgeons at medical spas might include nonsurgical procedures like chemical peels, microdermabrasion, Thermage or titan (which use radio frequency energy to heat the skin, which stimulates collagen production, tightening the skin), nonablative laser (stimulates collagen), and intense pulsed light that rejuvenates (website article[33]). I don't speak to Botox or fillers here because to me they do not make biologic sense. One is a neuromuscular poison; the other injects a substance from outside the body. I am certain this has worked for many, but it just doesn't pass the biologic test for me.

At a higher price, both literally and in the sense of invasiveness, there are many plastic surgery options. I have chosen not to talk about these, at least at this point, because I decided after starting my work with the aesthetician almost twelve years ago that I would subscribe to the Coco Chanel quote: "Nature gives you the face you have at twenty, it is up to you to merit the face you have at fifty." I have earned the face I have, including both the wrinkles I have and do not have; my face is the sum total of my life up to this point. Having earned the face, I am going to keep my wrinkles and lines, all the while minimizing them as much, and for as long, as possible! They tell the story of my life, my emotions, and my personal care. There are even website blogs, such as *Lines of Beauty* by Louise Cady Fernandes, which speak about aging gracefully one beautiful wrinkle at a time (website link[16]).

From my training and experience, I tend to agree with the thought from *The Aging Myth*[34] that we should be wary of [this doesn't mean rule out entirely] invasive cosmetic solutions because they are temporary, expensive, and [of course] invasive. *I think change that comes from natural, nonsurgical efforts is change that lasts.* This was certainly true in my experience treating gum disease.

Less talked about by aging experts I reviewed, I also believe in the power of wearing makeup for women. This is a very personal issue and a very personal decision, but for me it definitely works. I agree with *Wrinkle Free*[80] that it enhances others' perception of you; it strengthens your self-image; it makes you feel more socially secure; it lifts your mood; it produces a more positive outlook on life.

Wearing makeup is a lot like a good haircut. It can help you look and feel younger, according to WebMD (website article[36]), which suggests using primer and a light liquid foundation, a good magnifying mirror to avoid "clown eyes," eyeliner to enhance the shape of your eye, putting eyebrows back on if needed, avoiding lipstick bleeding into wrinkles, plumping lips with liner and lip-plumping lipstick, keeping lips moist, whitening stained teeth, getting good sleep and staying hydrated. The article also recommends wearing sunglasses to protect the delicate skin around your eyes and to keep you from squinting, making the most of your hair, exfoliating, using retinoids to reduce the appearance of fine wrinkles and fighting damage with antioxidants. Other suggestions included eating salmon for smoother skin (salmon comes up often, as you probably are noticing, which sure works for me up here in the Northwest), pampering your hands (as I said early on, I think they often are underestimated in the role they play in looking younger/older), not smoking, using sunscreen, and considering professional advice/help.

Last, but not least, there are some other tidbits of interesting information on aging that I came across that I hadn't thought about much but found thought-provoking. From *Forever Cool*:[70] "Quality fabrics can do a lot for aging skin." From *Beautiful Brain, Beautiful You*:[11] "Our face really does reflect how we feel and joy is a woman's [and man's] best cosmetic." From *The Aging Myth*:[34] "Our skin can mirror back to us where we are in terms of youth and vitality." I say, "Keep the wrinkles, but keep them to a minimum as much as possible."

SECTION 3: STAND UP AND BE COUNTED

I want to get old gracefully. I want to have good posture, I want to be healthy and be an example to my children.

—Sting

STOOPED OR STRAIGHT

I wholeheartedly agree and identify with this statement from Sting. It fits right in with aging gracefully and leaving a legacy, and yes, he is a boomer. Talking about posture, I hear those mothers' voices once again telling us that we should stand up or sit up straight. I remember this message going way back to my teen years, but as an adult, I stopped thinking about it much, until I started taking yoga classes and began looking around, taking note of my posture and that of others. What I noticed was that slumped shoulders or slouching are very aging and, as noted in *Beautiful Brain, Beautiful You*,[11] these portray an attitude of boredom (or acquiescence, or laziness).

But posture is a lot more than simply how we present ourselves and the impressions others get from it. This subject grabbed my attention during the research for this book, when I noted in *Change Your Age*[43] that pain, stiffness, and fatigue are the result of bad posture, movement, timing, and balance habits. Posture is a very strong reflection of how our major muscles and bones (our musculoskeletal structure) are aging. This is why our height gets measured during an annual physical. We need to pay close attention to this and do whatever we can to improve our posture and maintain our height.

As a return to the four steps we used to start this journey, stand sideways to the mirror and stare down those shoulders. Are they leaning forward toward the chest, or pulled back to line up with our ears? My yoga instructor has taught me that our shoulders should be lined up with our ears and our hips should be lined up with our shoulders, pulling our entire body into its natural, and intended, alignment. Not only is posture an important measure of our muscles and bones, it says a lot about how we feel physically, and how we feel emotionally.

Anti-Aging Quick Tip: According to WebMD, good posture is a quick and easy way to look better and several pounds thinner because slouching takes inches off your height and makes your stomach look rounder. (website article[18])

Goodness knows, most of us can benefit from several pounds thinner, so what can we do to improve the situation? Consider exercise, for one, since it strengthens bones and improves posture (*Beautiful Brain, Beautiful You*[11]). Consider concentration, for another, since paying attention (like Mother said) does actually help straighten those shoulders. It is very good news that we can improve posture by concentrating on it via body awareness[11] because, as promised, the goal here is to use practical information that is easy to incorporate into our lifestyle with minimal cost. Here is another perspective on the subject:

For good posture: rotate spine daily, check your posture at regular intervals,

*look in the mirror, practice standing
well at the supermarket line, walk tall by
looking ahead.*

(1001Ways to Stay Young Naturally[39])

I have a strong recommendation here based on my personal aging journey: incorporate yoga into your life somehow. Modern yoga is not religious, like some think. It is based upon five basic principles: positive thinking and meditation, proper relaxation, proper breathing, proper exercise, and proper diet.Yoga is a five-thousand-year-old practice that addresses flexibility, posture, breathing, balance, and strength. I have seen significant improvement in all these things since I began yoga. I started with one hour per week of beginner yoga, and after six months graduated to a second day of intermediate-level yoga. After two plus years, I value it even more than in the beginning because I have reaped many rewards for the time and effort spent.

Yoga benefits are extremely important as we age. In addition to improving posture, these practices help prevent falls through the balance and flexibility aspects, not to mention the "soothing" effects on the inner being and the opportunity for mindful (paying close attention to) introspection that it breeds, all of which are good for us. We will talk more about this when we discuss exercise in chapter 5 and what's good for our spirits in part 3.

SECTION 4: TO GROOM, TO BLOOM

If you have been taking care of yourself, you can expect to be graceful, attractive and youthful. There is absolutely no excuse not to be great-looking at sixty.

(Absolute Beauty[19])

Grooming may seem like small potatoes in the big picture of aging gracefully, but akin to what I said in the first impressions section about our smile and hair, I think its presence—or lack of, even more—speaks volumes about how we care for ourselves overall and how much we value taking care of our body. I like to think of it similar to the guru B. K. S. Iyengar: "The body is your temple. Keep it pure and clean for the soul to reside in." The things I ask myself in this area are: Are fingernails neat and clean? Was hand/body lotion used recently? When was the last shaving done? Was time taken for lip gloss or aftershave? Was makeup applied this morning? Is a magnifying mirror used for shaving, applying makeup, or removing unwanted hair? I mention these to get you thinking about the many little details of caring for the body and which ones are important to you.

Whatever we do each morning to prepare for our day is grooming. Our routines may be very individual, but the basis is the same: What are we willing to do to prepare the body for the journey of the day? Will we appear tired, dull, and unkempt, or will we sparkle and catch the attention of the fellow humans we meet during the day? This is simply another choice we make each day that influences the path we take.

Of course, with each choice there is a price to be paid (at a minimum, some time and effort), so the question is, is the price worth the outcome, as we talked about in the prologue. What is the ROI? Each of us must decide this, but I think grooming is a reflection of who we are and our attitude about how we want to portray ourselves to others and go through this life. It is like how we choose to decorate and keep our homes represents us to others. I try to choose the sparkle option at least a few times each week, depending on what's on my to-do list that day; i.e., housework and laundry? Maybe not. Lunch with a friend or a planned outing with my husband? Definitely.

I am luminous with age.

—Meridel Le Sueur

So those are my few words on grooming, but what about blooming? Another aspect of first impressions is about the blossoming of self related to our attitude toward aging. Our attitude shows in not only how we look but in how we behave. Do we see aging as an opportunity to bloom, without having to prove ourselves (*Prime Time: How Baby Boomers Will Revolutionize Retirement and Transform America*[24])? Are the challenges in our lives "sparkling moments" to change, experiment, push ourselves, and grow (*Forytude*[17])? Is our aging a new stage of even greater potential and strength, or "lost youth" (*Full Catastrophe Living*[2])? Are we present each moment and opening doors around us (*How We Age*[16])? Do we see that age brings a greater sense of mastery that serves as a source of pride and contributes to a positive self-image?[17]

People don't grow old. When they stop growing, they become old.

—Anonymous

Consider this: every effort we make, no matter how small, contributes to the overall picture of us! **Aging gracefully is a personal project and no one that has done it ever said it** would be easy, including Bette Davis, who once famously said: "Getting old isn't for sissies." But I WILL say that, with my personal experience and the aging knowledge I have gained, the results are worth the effort. We will visit this idea of attitude in more detail in the next chapter and in part 3.

SECTION 5: THE SHAPE WE'RE IN

It's never too late to become what you might have been.

—George Eliot

I'm not talking geometry here, but I am talking literal shape, and I am not talking about round being the shape. What is the waist measurement? What about the hips? **Do we know the value of our indices on body mass, or waist-to-height, or basal metabolic rate, or body fat and surface area, or Willoughby ideal weight and waist, to see what kind of shape the body is in?** (These can all be calculated with weight, height, waist, and age by visiting: http://home.fuse.net/clymer/bmi/.) Are we a giant apple, or a giant pear, or an extra-large from top to bottom? What shape are we now, and what shape do we want to be in?

Let's face it, the overall shape of the vessel also has a great deal of impact on how it is perceived, including the impression of how old it appears, not to mention the relationship between the shape we're in and aging well! This will get revisited in more detail in the exercise chapter, chapter 5. Remember how we started this journey with a 360-degree mirror evaluation (step four as we began)? Again, as the journey continues reevaluations are extremely important, in order to judge our progress and to take pride in that progress as we see visible improvement! This reevaluation includes how our shape is shaping up. Do we hear the battle cry? Do we hear our mothers' voices?

Baby Boomers know there is a possibility for a healthier, longer life span and [they] want to look the part.

(The DermaDoctor Skinstruction Manual[22])

PART 2:

THE INSIDE STORY

CHAPTER 1:

OUR PERSONAL CPU

SECTION 1: A THREE POUND UNIVERSE

The human brain has 100 billion nerve cells and each receives 100 messages per second. In the time it takes to read this sentence, brain cells have been doing more processing than the IRS's computer server.

(You Staying Young: The Owner's Manual for Extending Your Warranty[5])

Many of us vastly underestimate our brain, and take it for granted all too often, without thinking about it enough (pun intended)! Some have said that the human brain can do far more than we ever thought, and any limitations are imposed by us, not by any physical shortcomings of our brain (*Super Brain*[94]). In addition, I have learned from my research that much of the power of our brains is still not completely known or understood, so the potential is even greater than we know now in 2014.

But even at the potential we understand now, the human brain deserves a lot of respect. Not only does is have one hundred billion brain cells called neurons, but it has somewhere from a trillion to a quadrillion connections called synapses, which are in a constant, dynamic state of remodeling in response to the world around us.[94] It is an impressive, important organ that has been dubbed "the three-pound universe" because it both interprets and creates the world.[94] Our brain is astonishing, powerful, and the ultimate in sophistication. It is also one of the largest (skin, you may remember from the last chapter, is the largest) and more complex organs in the body.

A supercomputer's speed falls short compared to the human brain. Our brain has near-infinite storage and an astounding algorithm (a process or set of rules to be followed in calculations or other problem-solving operations, especially by a computer) to retrieve data, which scientists are still studying. I like to think of it as our personal central processing unit (CPU). Every second, every minute, all day and all night long, our brain is endlessly processing, regulating, sensing, creating, and recalling.

No matter which approach you take to anti-aging, our brain is involved.

(Super Brain[94])

With all of this power and potential, the brain is an important influencer on our aging pathway so it is important for our journey to understand generally how the brain works (the growing field of neuroscience) and the role it plays in our health, wellbeing, and aging. Dr. Eric R. Braverman, in *The Edge Effect*,[25] likens the way our brain interfaces with the body to the way an electrical outlet functions in our homes. To turn a light on, you plug in a lamp so that the electricity transfers from the house's circuitry to the lamp. In much the same way, the brain sends an electric current throughout our entire body, fueling our internal systems while maintaining our personality and orchestrating our health. I like this analogy. You could say the brain "lights" us up, or "turns us on"!

Orchestrating our health is obviously important to how we age. An entire field has developed to study this mind-body integrative medicine. This field has shown us the important role of our minds on health and disease (*Full Catastrophe Living*[2]). It is an approach to healing that honors the connections between the processes of the brain and the biological and biochemical reactions of the body. It harnesses the power of our thoughts and feelings to positively influence our physical health. This taps into the natural healing potential within each of us, which, as we talked about in the prologue, our bodies have more of than we probably realize. A question that begs an answer is how does it do that?

Did you know that brain function is based on chemistry? Our unique brain chemistry directly affects memory, attention, personality, and physical health, and *if you seem to be losing your edge, you are probably experiencing deficiencies in your brain biochemistry,* according to *The Edge Effect*[25]. The balanced brain slows aging, boosts energy, and is a path to weight loss, sexual vitality, clear thinking, a sharp memory, and more. (*RealAge: Are You as Young as You Can Be*[26]?)

I researched over one hundred books, and excerpted ninety-six, in addition to sixty-plus website articles for this manuscript. I actually purchased four of the books that I really connected with. One is *The Paleo Solution*,[15] which we will talk more about in chapter 3 and a second is Sanjay Gupta's book, *Chasing Life*[95] which we will also talk abut later. Another is *Super Brain*,[94] which we have been talking about. The third is *The Edge Effect*[25] by Dr. Eric Braverman, which we will talk about here. (I guess you can see that I am very interested in the brain!) Not only is the book great, if you are interested in lots of brain detail, but the author has developed a test that is in it (also available online) called the Braverman Nature Assessment Test. The test results show you what your dominant and deficient neurotransmitters are.

These neurotransmitters are the chemicals that travel along pathways in the brain, resulting in a variety of physical processes. They create unique electrical patterns that are transferred as brain waves (remember the light switch analogy?). Excesses of these biochemicals can flood synapses (connections) between brain cells, preventing signals from getting through to the next brain cell; if the neurotransmitters are deficient, the nerve signals may have nothing to travel on to make the connections that need to be made for our optimal well-being.

> Your unique brain chemistry [the combination of the neurotransmitters acetylcholine, dopamine, GABA, and serotonin] directly affects your memory, attention, personality and physical health. Deficiencies in these brain chemicals are the direct causes of many medical problems. Knowing how to restore deficiencies or imbalances is the way to regaining your "edge."
>
> (The Edge Effect[25])

Let's look at some specifics from *The Edge Effect* about the four neurotransmitters. Low dopamine increases cortisol (an internal body chemical messenger), which forces our metabolism to slow down and increases our appetite, plus causes bloating and weight gain around the midsection (an exceptionally bad combo); low levels of acetylcholine are linked to diabetes, Alzheimer's, and dementia; GABA creates a sense of calm and order (Zen), with low GABA being linked to emotional eating and excessive weight gain, and it is also associated with insulin resistance (according to Wikipedia, a condition where insulin becomes less effective at lowering blood sugar, which results in increased blood sugar, which can cause adverse health effects) and stress; serotonin allows the brain to recharge and rebalance with deep, restful sleep. The *Younger (Thinner) You Diet*[33] book, also by Dr. Eric Braverman, notes that low serotonin can contribute to lack of sleep, one of the great age accelerators. Taking the Braverman Test helps us sort out our balance and design our diets and lifestyle to give us back our edge. Like the RealAge tests and the Living to 100 Life Expectancy Test, I think this has tremendous value for our aging pathway.

We must dedicate ourselves to maintaining the fine chemical balance in our bodies.

(Retirement Is Not for Sissies[37])

LISTEN TO WHAT I SAY

An important part of brain function is communication. The mind expresses itself through the body, which becomes the messenger to the person within, as well to those around us (*Body Odyssey*[83]). Our soma speaks to us. Are we listening? Do we "hear" our thoughts? This is important because our thoughts literally make a difference in our aging pathway, both inwardly and outwardly (*Age Proof Your Body*[47]). We will consider this internal communication with our body a number of times throughout the book.

Part of what we communicate to those around us is attitude, another important brain-centered influencer on aging. From *Younger Next Year*:[36] "You can, just as easily, make up your mind—and tell your body—to live as if you were fifty, maybe even younger, for most of the rest of your life." My sister, Janice, and I have always been very close, being only one year plus six days apart in age and having always shared a room while growing up. When I told her about this book and asked her what she thought was a major factor in aging, she volunteered right away that she felt attitude was a big deal in aging gracefully. This has been echoed by many of the aging authorities whose material I have reviewed.

Anti-Aging Quick Tip: "Those of us who have a generally positive attitude toward aging live longer than those who do not." (*The Longevity Bible*[42])

Age Proof Your Body[47] says: "If you want to live vitally and long...choose to think youthfully and be playful. If you plan to live a long life, be prepared to work on your attitude." I agree completely with the crucial role of attitude. Aging gracefully takes getting up with a fighting but positive attitude, then thinking young and playful, eating right, getting some exercise, keeping stress under control, avoiding "bad" habits, finding challenges to conquer, keeping a social network close by—oh, and did I remember to say brushing and flossing daily (discussed in chapter 1 to a much greater extent than would probably be called "normal")?

If you want to live to be 100 or older, you can't just sit around waiting for it to happen. You have to get up each day and go for it!

—George Burns

> **Anti-Aging Quick Tip: We can think ourselves young by thinking youthful thoughts.**

Maybe part of how a positive attitude helps us live longer has to do with how that positive thinking feeds back to our body. *Grow Younger, Live Longer*[53] tells us that: "Fresh and youthful thoughts create fresh and youthful molecules." I am very excited here, as I do believe, based on my long career in healthcare and on the research for this book, that we can "think ourselves young" because of the vast potential our brains have to continue to develop, which is unique to the human species.

Man is the only animal to have been granted the ability to continue developing during the later periods of life...It is incumbent on us to use this ability.

(The Art of Aging[52]*)*

Those fresh and youthful molecules indicate regenerative ability. *Super Brain*[94] states that the brain has amazing healing powers and our ability to rewire our brains remains intact from birth to the end of life. "In fact, the brain contains stem cells that are capable of maturing into new brain cells throughout life." This is an important piece to the aging gracefully puzzle. It makes complete biologic sense to me; this important central organ is made to last *at least* as long as the soma within which it resides. Nature would not have it be otherwise.

Knowing that we can rewire and heal our brain from birth to the end leads us to the conclusion that the old adage that you can't teach old dogs new tricks is false. *Beautiful Brain, Beautiful You*[11] says that even if we have neglected our brain for years, it won't hold a grudge! The potential is always there.

Not only can old dogs learn new tricks, we must learn them to stay fully alive.

(Retirement Is Not for Sissies[37])

In addition, there is this from *The Wisdom Paradox*:[84] "Not only is it possible for a vigorous mental life to continue throughout the whole lifespan, but also in some people it actually reaches its peak at a rather advanced age." **Older does not mean we don't still have powerful minds.** Our brain might actually hit its highest point in our later life. *The Mature Mind*[30] tells us that healthy older brains are robust with more potential than we realize. Let's talk now about how we can enhance and capitalize on that potential.

BRAIN CALISTHENICS

Because our brains play such a key role, quality longevity obviously requires taking care of our CPU so if healthy aging is a goal, we have to be responsible for keeping it in good working order. As part of that obligation/opportunity, it is essential to the brain that we maintain blood flow and avoid chronic inflammation. The flip side is, we must avoid brain burglars (they compromise blood flow and/or promote inflammation, paving the way for stroke), which are high blood pressure, high cholesterol, high blood sugar, obesity, abdominal fat, and smoking (*Beautiful Brain, Beautiful You*[11]). We will talk in more detail about this in the next chapter.

> **Anti-Aging Quick Tip: Challenging our brain not only keeps the brain in peak shape, it actually enhances the brain's performance.**

Besides having brain essentials and avoiding brain burglars, there is another aspect to taking care of our brains and how our brains are part of our aging pathway. The brain, like the rest of our body, fares best if we use it in a way that stimulates it. Your brain isn't a muscle, but it still needs to be exercised to achieve peak performance; i.e., use it or lose it (*The Everything Anti-Aging Book*[55]). Yet, it is really more than "use it or lose it," because using the brain in a way that challenges it can actually *enhance* the circuitry and performance, according to brain experts. Not only that, but using it may be key to keeping it healthy, again paralleling the rest of our body and making perfect biologic sense. Think about that idea for a second as you consider this extremely important bit of expert aging advice:

The more we are engaged in stimulating activities, the less likely we are to develop dementia.

(Beautiful Brain, Beautiful You[11]*)*

I think my professional career was good for my brain: doing thousands of microsurgeries (surgery done with magnification), teaching, lecturing, and publishing papers for the last thirty years, not to mention running my own business by myself during that time—playing the role of CEO, COO, CFO, personnel director and marketing VP all at once—while also doing my surgeon job each day! This book has been good for my brain, too (and the rest of me, for sure), since I read and think, then I write, then I read and think some more, then I rewrite, etc. Writing this book has also stimulated my brain by having to learn a lot of new tricks in Microsoft's Word software, such as setting up a table of contents that updates automatically as the document changes. Overall, I have found that the learning curve for computer software programs and technological devices is somewhat to extensively challenging and therefore they are brain-enhancing. We certainly live at the right time to take advantage of this since there is so much out there that it is hard to keep track of it all.

So we know we need to use it, but what are some other options besides technology? There are as many options as there are brains to think of them. Here, as an example, is one aging expert's take on maintaining our brain power:

To maintain cognitive function:

* *Exercise memory.*
* *Stimulate your brain with puzzles.*
* *Read.*
* *Take continuing education (CE).*
* *Teach CE.*
* *Learn a foreign language.*

- *Start a hobby that requires coordination like dancing, painting, or a musical instrument.*
- *Do math calculations in your head.*
- *Write your autobiography.*

(The Everything Anti-Aging Book[55])

Let's consider these further. Many of them involve education/ learning. We are designed to be continuous, lifetime learners, and lifelong learning gives our brain a reason to function (*You Staying Young: The Owner's Manual for Extending Your Warranty[5]*). I love that as I have loved school and learning since kindergarten. Another aging authority said that the key to staying young is in part learning whatever and whenever you can (Aging Abundantly on Facebook). That resonates with me. Learning as a lifelong adventure to help us keep our brain power sounds awesome and I can definitely relate to this perspective:

I am learning all the time. The tombstone will be my diploma.

—*Eartha Kitt*

An important activity for life-long learning is reading. Reading is good for our brains because it expands our knowledge and gives our brains a great workout (*Beautiful Brain, Beautiful You*[11]). I am thrilled with that! Let there be books, books, and more books! Reading is one of my favorite brain-stimulating activities. I have been in love with books since I was six, sitting in an apple tree dreaming of having my own library.

Books allow us to travel far and wide, to find ourselves in all types of venues, without ever leaving our recliner! Reading satisfies our curiosity about the world we **don't** live in every day, as well as expands our view of the one we do live in. The feel of a good book in my hands, turning the crisp pages (I don't see myself ever being much of an e-book reader for this reason), is not only good for the brain, I know now that it is good for the whole me. It is also relaxing for me, which as we will see in chapter 5, is also excellent for our aging pathway. I once saw an uncredited post on Facebook that said something to the effect that if you have a library and a garden, you have everything you need. I think so.

Curiosity is the cure for boredom. There is no cure for curiosity.

—Dorothy Parker

Books, reading, and learning are closely linked to curiosity, which I think is also extremely important to our brains and to aging well. "Our brains are built to feed our curiosity, our urge to discover, uncover, and invent" (from a PBS special, "Hopeful Aging"). As said in *The Art of Aging*,[52] it [curiosity] has a driven character to it. At least for myself, inquisitiveness about the world definitely drives me intellectually, providing motivation to expand myself by expanding my knowledge as I learn new things. And to think how well we are treating our brain and our aging by cozying down with a good book in pursuit of what intrigues us!

From a more global perspective, *Keep Your Brain Young*[54] notes that there are three factors characterizing those who maintained their mental abilities over time:

1. *Mentally active.*

2. *Physically active.*

3. *They maintained a sense of effectiveness in the world around them, a sense of control over their lives, and they felt they were contributing.*

One way to be mentally active and challenge our brain is the use of neurobics (mental exercises designed to create new neural pathways in the brain by using the senses in unconventional ways, which strengthens the brain's natural affinity for learning new things); i.e., accomplish ordinary tasks in new ways by using all five senses. Some examples of this from *Looking After Your Body: An Owner's Guide to Successful Aging*[56] and others include: crossing the room with our eyes closed at night without turning on the lights, or getting dressed with our eyes closed, or writing with our nondominant hand, or brushing our teeth with our nondominant hand. (I do this one several times a week—what a surprise!)

Anti-Aging Quick Tip: Doing everyday tasks with our nondominant hand can definitely pay off in terms of not only strengthening the brain, but it might really come in "handy" should we ever lose the use of our dominant one.

Back in the early '80s, I heard someone talking about how valuable being ambidextrous is, especially as we grow older. This is neurobics. They recommended starting with simple tasks such as brushing our hair with the nondominant hand, or opening a door, or, as noted above, brushing our teeth. I made this part of my life, and down the road a few years, I was even able to suture

with my left hand, even though I am clearly right-hand dominant. Imagine the advantages if we ever have a stroke! I think
this is way worth the struggle and effort it takes to achieve the
very valuable short-term and long-term benefits. The return on
investment could be enormous!

Other aging experts talk about what's good for our brains
in other terms, including the value of improving our awareness
(knowledge or perception of a situation) and mindfulness (staying
focused in the present). One authoritative source noted the following: brain "pleasers" include teaching, living in the moment
(mindfulness), and improving awareness; for example, thinking
about every tooth as you brush it (*You Staying Young: The Owner's
Manual for Extending Your Warranty*[5]).

With consideration for staying focused on the present and
our mental well-being, *The Longevity Bible*[42] says that mindfulness provides us efficiency in mental tasks; perseverance builds
learning memory; focusing on details helps us retain longer; and
curiosity expands our mental horizons. *Super Brain*[94] combines
mindfulness with memory: a mindful memory program would
include being passionate about your life and the experiences you
fill it with, enthusiastically learning new things, paying attention to things you want to remember later, understanding that
most memory lapses are actually learning lapses, and actively
retrieving older memories and relying less on memory crutches
like lists. Mindful memory also includes expecting to keep our

memories intact, not blaming or fearing occasional lapses, understanding that if a memory doesn't come right away, we don't need to consider it lost (give the brain's retrieval system some time), and being wide-ranging in our mental activities.[94] I think that this mindfulness/awareness is another important part of our aging gracefully pathway. *Super Brain*[94] puts this spin on it: awareness contains the power to transform our world.

Interestingly, besides our CPU needing stimulation, there is some evidence that to keep our memory young, the brain may also need downtime to process information and consolidate memories. In addition, less noise and more silence, less artificial light and more natural light, less stuffy air and more fresh breaths outdoors, and less clutter and more wide-open spaces may also help keep our brain closer to age eighteen (website article[48]).

ADVANTAGE AGE

Last, but not least, there are some significant advantages to aging where our brain is concerned. Our lifelong learning, curiosity and whatever brain "pleasers" or activities we do all contribute to our wisdom and competence, which can only be achieved by experience, and therefore *years* of living. Wisdom distinguishes, and is unique to, the elder segment of our society. "Wisdom is the precious gift of aging" (*The Wisdom Paradox*[84]). It also dictates constant reevaluation of ourselves—rethinking all we have been, all that we are, and all that we can be, no matter the age (*The Art of Aging*[52]). Competence, which is another reward of aging, is our ability to do a job well; a combination of knowledge, skills, and behavior that improves performance.[84] Youth may have vim and vigor, but we ageds may have a leg up with our smarts and skills! We will talk more about this in part 3, chapter 1.

SECTION 2: FEED YOUR HEAD

Lean into life, fill ourselves with rich experiences while challenging our minds and supporting our brains.

(Winning at Aging[44]*)*

Grace Slick shouts: "Feed your head!" Well, I don't know that she was talking about stimulating our brains with actual food, or reading or puzzles, or doing unfamiliar tasks, but I think she was "right on." We need both literal and figurative "fuel" for our minds. We talked about figurative brain food in the prior section. Let's mix in some of the literal. Did you know that patients with Alzheimer's disease have lower ascorbate (a derivative of vitamin C) levels in their blood, and that animal studies have shown vitamins C and E interacting with each other improved performance in certain memory tests (website article[38])? Or did you know that berries are good for the brain, according to a study that suggests the fruits can help fend off the mental decline of aging (website article[39])? *Or did you know that a human study showed that vitamin D, together with curcumin (found in turmeric spice), appeared to stimulate the immune system in a way that helped clear the brain of toxic amyloid beta* (**website article**[10])*?* I am thinking poached salmon dressed with herbs and sweet potato fries sprinkled with turmeric!

> **Anti-Aging Quick Tip: Use turmeric and other spices, along with eating lots of fruits and vegetables, not only to spice things up taste-wise, but to help avoid cognition problems.**

I have said before but will say again: pay real attention to this turmeric. My gut instinct says there is really something to this, because it kept coming up over and over again as I researched the literature out there on aging. But turmeric isn't the only "brain" spice. According to the author of *Younger (Thinner) You Diet*,[33] there are several brain-accelerating spices: allspice, basil, cumin, peppermint, sage, thyme, and turmeric. In addition, the scent of cinnamon enhances cognitive processing, including attention, memory, and visual-motor speed (*Ageless Face, Ageless Mind*[21]). And the great news is, the spices taste and smell wonderful, so they are good for our senses, too, which is good for our brain. Seems like a win-win all around to me, and I have definitely adopted these into my lifestyle like never before. I would much rather use turmeric or peppermint than take a pill of some kind. I highly recommend making use of these "spicy" aging tidbits!

Another brain food flash: eating your veggies isn't only about the heart anymore. A laboratory has shown that eating a diet containing fruits and vegetables high in antioxidant activity will show similar benefits to the brain with respect to aging as has been shown in the heart. Lead scientist James Joseph says:

> *Those who regularly consume sufficient quantities of fruits and vegetables have 40 percent less risk of developing Alzheimer's disease.*
>
> *(website article[9])*

According to the CEO of Food for the Brain Foundation (website article[40]), an article published by two leading neuroscientists concluded that "successful brain ageing [*sic*] is possible for most individuals if they maintain healthy diets and lifestyles throughout their adult life." Learning new things, having good social contact, having a sense of purpose, exercising, eating more fish, chocolate, red wine (within limits), and green tea are a few of the factors that reduce the risk of memory decline, according to the article. AARP's website shared the following ideas for brain foods: go Mediterranean (which has also been supported by *Food for the Brain E-News*, as noted above), cut back on red meat and dairy, ramp up foods with omega-3s, binge on blueberries, slash trans fats, take the salt shaker off the table, and reduce sugar and simple carbs (website article[57]). And get this: cocoa has potent neuroprotective effects, protecting brain cells from inflammation. It also upsets the wrinkle-producing process (*Forever Young*[71]). Who would have thought?

Other aging experts have shared lists, including both literal and figurative food for the brain tidbits such as the following from *1001 Ways to Stay Young Naturally*,[39] some of which we have already considered.

Brain Food

- Cook with sage (especially purple).
- Take ginkgo.
- Use your "wrong" hand to do things.

- *Be a lifelong student.*
- *Learn a language.*
- *Meditate daily.*
- *Try balancing postures.*
- *Enjoy family and friends.*
- *Dine on fish.*
- *Eat greens.*
- *Try green and black teas.*
- *Unplug the phone.*
- *Play games.*
- *Walk backward and sideways to forge new circuits in the brain.*
- *Walk, don't drive.*
- *Take the stairs.*
- *Work in the yard.*
- *Harness the urge for spring cleaning or clearing clutter; scrub floors, paint walls.*

LET'S MAKE SOME SENSE OF IT

Our senses (sight, hearing, touch, smell, taste), and keeping them working well, is also part of brain function and the kind of well-being that helps us age as gracefully as possible.

Protecting our senses is important, since there is a direct relationship between your senses (the brain creating the opportunity to "sense") and the health and well-being of our bodies (*SuperHealth*[59]).

There are foods that are specifically good for your senses, including pomegranates, blueberries, walnuts, spinach, kiwis, oranges, wheat germ, and almonds ([59]). You can also take a RealAge Eye Test (website link[3]) to evaluate the health of your eyes and to check your risk of three major eye problems. Advice and an assessment for hearing and information on changes in taste or smell can also be found on this website.

Stimulating our senses is also good for our brain (which is good for aging in general), and we can use sense-specific mental exercises to do this. For example, "You can improve your vision by exercising your eyes. Brain Gym offers a set of exercises designed to stimulate vision, memory, reading and coordination" www.braingym.org (*The Body Knows How to Stay Young*[64]).

Anti-Aging Quick Tip: Enjoy music, smell a fragrant flower, or savor the taste of a favorite food and reap well-being rewards for your brain.

We can stimulate our other senses by "stopping to smell the roses," listening to good music, savoring the taste of food in our mouths (which is good for digestion), etc. I have a personal theory that we can stimulate *and* protect our senses by challenging them. For instance, I purposely turn the TV volume down low so that I have to work at hearing. I close my eyes to smell and try to describe the smell to myself. I also resist wearing my glasses for reading unless I really cannot read what I am seeing. I think you see (ha, good one) what I mean.

SECTION 3: STRESSING THE POINT

Stress is not what happens to us. It's our response to what happens. And response is something we can choose.

—Maureen Killoran

We will talk more about stress when we cover our aging enemies, but I want to begin the conversation here as we discuss our brain because our brain orchestrates our response to anything that challenges us, including any stress we are confronted with.

You may already know that chronic stress ages us, but did you know that it physically damages the brain because cortisol (our stress hormone) can kill neurons (brain cells) in the memory center (*Beautiful Brain, Beautiful You*[11])? This is very important and very powerful knowledge.

To live long, it is necessary to live slowly.

—Cicero

So, managing stress is another very potent key to our brain aging well and for us to live a long, healthy, happy life. But our daily lives are full of various stressors and they have to be dealt with somehow. Therein lies the rub! How can we do it? Well, I don't have any training in cognitive behavioral psychology, but I have been told it is a matter of reframing. I myself used a variety of strategies to deal with the stress of being a surgeon, business owner, lecturer, author, etc. I had interests outside of work that I found relaxing, like hiking, rock climbing, skiing, music, even trashy romance novels.

Exercise was, and still is, a big stress releaser for me, which is a great motivator to keep at it, with the value added reward of being healthier. I also learned early on how important it was to leave work at work. In my mind, I used the image of flipping the light switch as I left the office to keep the intensity of it there, acting out one of my small group of dogma not to take work home.

Luckily, good friends had also warned me when I was new in practice not to let periodontics run my life, but to have interests outside of my field. This helped me disconnect from that very big stressor in my life early in the game. Each of us will have to find the things that work for us, but finding them is very important to longevity and healthy aging! We need to deal with it to protect our brain. If how stress damages the brain by killing neurons doesn't "grab" you, consider this:

Distressed people are 2–4x more likely to develop Alzheimer's.

(Beautiful Brain, Beautiful You[11])

But, because stress keeps us "wired" and "spinning," there never seems to be time to relieve or reduce stress—**wrong way, U-turn, flip!** The wear and tear on us is much too big a price to pay. We *must* make the time, even if it is simply a hot bath before bed, a good book while relaxing in the recliner, or some meditation. Find a way that works for you on a frequent, if not daily, basis. By the way, did you know that meditation aids healing because of its powerful calming effect on the body that neutralizes the disabling effects of stress (*Age Proof Your Body*[47])? We will consider this further in part 3, chapter 1.

A stress-reliever that works well for me now in my postperiodontist years is digging in the dirt in the garden. There is nothing like tilling the soil and watching the results of those efforts as they come to fruition to give us a sense of connectedness and relaxation, not to mention the good stuff for our senses (like the sweet smell of lilacs on a warm, sunny day in May, or the bright taste of a freshly-picked tomato in July), and the healthy nutrition it provides! Reading a good book, which we know is good for our brain, can also be very calming, as it transports us out of our "real" world. Some books may even put us to sleep. OMG, I hope not this one! We will talk a lot more about things that have calming effects in chapter 5.

To wrap up our personal CPU discussion, let's recap the high points: understand and value the brain; think positive; exercise the brain; take age advantage of wisdom and competence; eat foods good for the brain; stimulate and protect the senses; and de-stress to protect the brain.

CHAPTER 2:

TURNING BACK THE AGING CLOCK

SECTION 1: WILL THE REALAGE STAND UP?

First off, let me start with another one of my collection of dogma that I have latched on to over the years as a health-care provider. I personally don't think a prosthetic device or replacement organ is ever as good as the nature-made version! I don't care if it's a tooth, a heart, or a knee, hip, or arm. Man-made is not as good, even with the best of minds, hands, hearts, and intentions. With my almost 40 years of experience in health care spanning from my pre-dental years as a hygienist to the end of my clinical periodontal practice, I have concluded that it is always better to keep the nature-made version if at all possible—or at least for as long as possible! I truly don't think we will ever do better than the parts and pieces that we came into this world with.

I do not say this lightly. I don't like and don't subscribe to much dogma because it is too inflexible, and that is exactly the opposite of biologic systems, which are very fluid and flexible. There are most certainly things that I am unaware of, and who knows what the future will bring, but from my vantage point, I do believe it represents the here and now accurately.

The exquisite construction, wiring, heating/cooling, plumbing, etc., of our bodies is beyond our ability to duplicate. Our bodies are such fine-tuned machines with such fascinating and precise interplay and effectiveness that it is nothing short of astonishing! I find words very limiting when I try to tell you how amazing I think it truly is. Although there is some disagreement about the exact source of our sophisticated human form, I think we can all agree that the outcome is excellence beyond excellent. If you want to be really impressed, try studying human physiology. You will never be the same again when it comes to how you think about the human body. Enough said. If you can pardon me for and accept my dogma, then the next logical thought is that we must try to keep our bodies and our body parts as "young" as we can so they last us as long as possible, so that we don't need, or can at least minimize the need, to resort to the man-made ones. This also keeps us younger in total.

You are only as young as your oldest part.

——Dr. Eric Braverman, The Edge Effect[25]

Turning back the aging clock is what this chapter, and the remaining three chapters in part 2, are all about. We will begin here in section 1 with some baseline general concepts/ideas/tips, followed by delving deeper into the detail and specifics in sections 2 and 3, and the chapters beyond. My overriding purpose remains the same: to filter out and share knowledge that gives us practical, biologically sound advice on aging from aging experts because, as we have said before, knowledge is power, and understanding how our body ages gives us the power to help us select the tools we individually need to age gracefully. No longer will we need to take my mother's sisters' approach to age: trying to fool others by telling untruths about being younger than we actually are. With effort and choices based on understanding, we will be able to speak the truth, which will be about our biologic real age being less than our most recent birthday age. Yahoo! "Celebrate good times, come on!"

TESTING, TESTING

I would strongly recommend putting this book down at this point to take the time to complete the free RealAge Test on RealAge.com (website link[3]) before you read on. RealAge.com is one of three or four of my favorite healthy lifestyle websites, and their test is all about turning back the aging clock. It covers four major areas in the following order: health, feelings, diet, and fitness. Similar to the RealAge site health test, this chapter covers the internal battles for health that we fight in the aging war. Chapters to follow will cover the other three major areas. Taking the test before continuing this book will create the opportunity for the reader to gain even more out of the bits of expert aging advice herein because it will establish a foundational basis for their application to each of us as unique individuals.

The RealAge Test is very thorough, taking you through questions about all the potential "influencers" on aging. It results in a number that represents our real age, which is a quick, scientific calculation of how young or old our body actually is. All the information that is part of the RealAge name is held up to stringent scientific review, so it meets the biologically sound criteria. Once we complete the test, we also get an action plan to grow younger; i.e., what areas could benefit from change that would lead to a younger us, turning that clock back. We cannot beat that kind of help at any cost (which is our time only, in this case), and I think it is really worth the ROI to do it. Speaking of cost, one of my favorite concepts (my wording and I shared this in the prologue) from one of my mentors, Dr. Saul Schluger, is this: no matter our choices, there will always be a price to be paid. The question we have to ask, and answer, is, will the outcome be worthy of the price. If it is, it makes sense to do it. If the outcome is not worthy of the price, then we need to choose another path. So when I talk about ROI (return on investment) throughout this book, this is my basis for making and considering that calculation.

I took the RealAge Test the first time about four years ago, and have updated it a number of times since. It has been an excellent barometer for my battle with aging, and I find it both motivating and informative. Learning our real age can be very humbling. The flip side is, as we make progress, it can also be very rewarding and exciting; for example, to tell someone my biologic age is 54.7 when the actual chronologic age is nearly sixty-two, a difference of just shy of eight years! Or to find out my mouth age is thirty-seven at sixty-two, or that my skin age is forty-six at sixty-two, or that my knees and hips are only thirty-two at sixty-two.

I think you can see that this is a wonderful tool for goal setting and benchmarking successes to celebrate. (And please don't forget to celebrate!) Imagine if we could all go around telling our several years younger real age versus our calendar age or our mouth age instead of our birthday age. For those who might be looking for a mate, imagine the value of those biologic age results when you knock some significant years off your last birthday age! Well, at least those whose real age is smaller than their chronologic age would want to strut about it...but we can ALL strive for that end result if we want to!

Now, with the knowledge of our how old our body thinks we are, we can move forward with turning back the clock, starting with a big-picture perspective by asking this question: What kind of relationship do we have with our body? We discussed mindfulness, awareness, and mind-body integration in the prior chapter when we talked about the brain. We noted then that our body does talk to us to tell us what is happening with our inner selves.

Let's ask some specific personal questions about that. Are you aware of your body sending you signals about how it is doing? How much are you in tune with those subtle messages your body sends? When did you last check in with your body parts? For example, if you have had heartburn, what did that tell you about your stomach/digestion, and how might you have used that information?

Or, when was the last time you thought about the role the mouth and chewing plays in starting the digestive process, or took note of how your GI tract is functioning, or not functioning, as the case may be? Do you ever take note of your heart rate and ask, what is this telling me? Or, do you ever check in with your body and ask, what is the rhythm of my breathing saying about me and where I am at this moment? Do you hear what I hear?

Anti-Aging Quick Tip: Listening to what our body tells us helps us use our anti-aging tools in an optimal way.

Do you take your blood pressure at home at various times of the day and under various conditions to really get an accurate measure, and then ask, what does this mean to me? By the way, last year my internist told me that some research has shown that blood pressure readings taken at home are much more accurate than those taken at the doctor's office. I know that this "white coat syndrome" is definitely true for me, as the stress of worrying about what my blood pressure reading will be during my annual physical sends my blood pressure soaring, so I now take a list of recent readings of my own to the appointment. All this talk about listening to our body may sound silly or like "overkill" to some of the readers, but it is actually, in my opinion, not silly at all. Instead, it is of paramount importance and is generally vastly underused and underestimated. As said so well in *Super Brain*,[94] *the most personalized approach to longevity is tuning in to our bodies, i.e., self-awareness.*

Re-establish your relationship with your
body parts by recalling their function.

(Fortytude[17])

To understand and win the fight against aging, we need to have a basic understanding of, and a relationship with, our body parts and their function. Exactly like we need to check in with ourselves in a mirror, we need to keep in touch with that part of ourselves we cannot see and listen to any information/feedback we get. This information is very valuable, and can really help us use our anti-aging tools at an optimal level and age more gracefully, not to mention improving our longevity.

TO CHOOSE, OR NOT TO CHOOSE, THAT IS THE QUESTION

This tuning in to hear our bodies' messages is an important aging choice we can make for a more graceful aging pathway. In fact, the composition of all the choices we make, and don't make, every day and how those choices affect our bodies determines our aging pathway. As we learned in part 1, chapter 1, genetics only accounts for about one-third of the factors that lead to a long life—the remaining *majority* **two-thirds** is about the choices we make every moment, every day: what we eat or drink; what we do or don't do; whether we have a smoke, or not; what time we go to bed and get up, etc. You get the idea. We can choose to live healthier and therefore longer and there is even genetic testing available now to help with that. A company by the name of Interleukin Genetics offers the Personal Inherent Health Genetic Testing Service, which has a series of four health and wellness tests available to empower us and help prevent some of the chronic diseases of aging through diet and lifestyle recommendations based on insights from a trusted source of genetic research.

The tests include a weight management test, a heart health test, a nutrition test, and a bone health test. When I took these genetics tests, I found out that I absorb more dietary fat and have a slower metabolism, and that I am more responsive to high-intensity exercise, so if I want to lose weight, I have to cut fat intake and get in some thirty-minute-plus cardio sessions each week. I also learned that I do not have increased risk of postmenopausal bone loss; I have efficient vitamin B metabolism, but suboptimal management of oxidative stress, so I need more antioxidants compared to those who don't have this genetic variant; and I have low risk level for having a heart attack due to genetic factors. Like the numerous tests offered on RealAge.

com, this is fabulously useful information for fine-tuning my aging pathway!

This is another example of a tool available to us to empower us with knowledge about aging and longevity if we make the choice to use it. From a website article[16] came the following ten more "every day" examples of other choices that we might make to live longer and healthier (please take special note of number five):

1. Quit Smoking: adds +four to eight years.

2. Cut Out Fast Food: adds +four years.

3. Get Moving: adds +two to four years.

4. Shed Those Pounds: adds +three to four years.

5. Floss Your Pearly Whites: adds +six years

6. Take A Break From Work: adds +two years.

7. Flex Your Brain: adds +two years.

8. Snack Smarter: adds +two to six years.

9. Stay In Bed Longer: adds +two years.

10. Have More Sex: adds +three to eight years.

As discussed in the previous chapter and, not surprisingly, our attitude also plays a role in how we age. As reported on the *Refined by Age* blog, research by Becca Levy proves that having a positive outlook on aging can add seven and a half years to one's life. "Positive affirmations about ourselves and our aging process are very important to our overall health and wellness" (website blog[62]).

The book *RealAge: Are You as Young as You Can Be?*[26] supports the concept of choices by saying: place a value on your daily choices; e.g., stairs versus elevator or apple versus cookie to lower your real age. "Stay young—for the rest of your life[26]."

Anti-Aging Quick Tip: RealAge.com (website link[3])provides these examples about choices and aging: Two twenty-minute walks per day can take five years off your biologic age. Regularly wearing your seat belt and driving within five miles per hour of the speed limit can make you 3.4 years younger. If you avoid periodontal disease by brushing and flossing, it makes your RealAge 6.4 years younger.

By now I am sure that this will come as a great shock to all, but—surprise, surprise—I am *absolutely* on board with that last one! In addition, the book[26] lists important age reducers and healthy habits (choices we repeat over and over) to keep us young:

Age reducers: antioxidants (oxidation is body's equivalent of "rusting"), calcium and vitamin D, vitamin C, a balanced diet, maybe vitamin E, foliate.

Healthy habits to keep you young: sleep well, eat breakfast, drink alcohol moderately, and own a furry friend.

AGING FACTORS AND ACCELERATORS

A good place to begin this part of our discussion, I think, is to look at a global picture, focusing on the categories of important aging factors used by *RealAge*.[26] We will then "funnel" down and look at more specific aging accelerators and how they actually damage our bodies as we age. At the end of the chapter, and sprinkled in here and there beforehand, we will look at some general strategies to fight back, getting into more detail about that in chapters 3 and beyond. Using this framework is helpful, I feel, because it allows us to digest the material in chunks instead of all at once.

RealAge[26] shares with us what they think are the three most important factors that affect aging: aging of the arteries, social/environmental factors, and aging of the immune system. There has been a lot of discussion in the last few years about the first two factors, so we won't spend a great many words here. Instead, we will highlight a few aging tidbits to refresh our memory and get us thinking globally about the subject. For example: for the heart, we need regular exercise; and it is important not to become sedentary (*Healthy At 100*[14]). We need to slow arterial aging, keep our blood pressure at 115/76 or lower, some of us need to take daily aspirin, some may need to do hormone replacement therapy, and we all need to watch our weight and what we eat to protect our heart and arteries ([26]). We will talk a lot more about eating well in chapter 3.

Approximately 30 illnesses and diseases are linked to being overweight, including cardiovascular (heart) disease, high blood pressure, strokes, diabetes, arthritis, and sleep apnea and strokes.

(Healthy Aging for Dummies[81])

With regard to reducing social/environmental hazards to improve longevity, *RealAge*[26] offers this aging well advice, along with others:

> *Don't smoke, use safety to prevent accidents, wear seat belts and helmets, try to reduce exposure to toxic chemicals, enjoy sex, don't use drugs.*

Perhaps not as commonly talked about is the very important role of the immune system and how that built-in shield against illness and disease plays a role in aging. To function properly, our immune system must detect a wide variety of agents, from viruses to parasitic worms, and distinguish them from our own healthy tissue (Wikipedia definition). Degeneration of our immune system is one of the more important consequences of accumulated aging damage, and as our system becomes weakened, disease becomes a much greater threat and our cancer risk rises (website article[46]). Like other parts of our bodies, there are things we can do to help our immune system.

Anti-Aging Quick Tip: We need to laugh often; it is so very good for us!

Livestrong.com gives this advice: wash your hands regularly, keep yourself hydrated, quit smoking, get enough vitamin D, exercise, sleep well, and laugh often (website link[1]). RealAge.com (website link[3]) talks about weight loss to strengthen our immune system; reducing stress; and certain foods we can eat to enhance our immune system, such as kiwi fruit, pistachios, mushrooms, and grape juice, along with tea. We will expand on this subject when we talk a little about general battle strategies at the end of this chapter.

Anti-Aging Quick Tip: Drink water to be healthy, think clearly, and even lose weight.

Before we leave off talking about the important factors that affect aging, and go forward with a discussion about more specific aging accelerators, I want to add one last very key concept about a broadly influential factor that affects how our body ages. It came up often in my research and has been talked about in **many** venues: whether we drink enough water, or not, has a powerful influence on our internal (and external, meaning skin) well-being and aging. "More than 2/3 of the weight of the human body is water. The brain is over 95% water. Your blood is 82%

water. Your lungs are 90% water. Your muscle tissue contains 73% water" (*Healthy Aging for Dummies*[81]).

All systems and organs require water to function. You can't last more than few days without water, a few weeks without food.

(Transcend: Nine Steps to Living Well Forever[9]*)*

Drinking enough liquid can increase concentration, energize your body, maximize your immune system, help prevent constipation, rehydrate the skin, and lower the risk of developing gallstones, kidney stones, and even bladder cancer (*Natural Health at 50*[72]). The hard part about drinking a lot of water is logistics. It is a bonafide struggle, in part because it keeps us near a bathroom about an hour or two after drinking a glass. I try hard, but this is one that I battle with at times. So, why is the struggle worth the price we pay for it? How does the ROI evaluation come out? If the previous reasons are not motivational enough, consider the following on water's purpose:

To replenish what's been lost to perspiration and respiration. To flush toxins.

To keep you body's care temperature balanced.
To help keep the blood circulating.

(Healthy Aging for Dummies[81])

That last one is certainly very important to our soma's life span, which we have learned is a brain essential in addition to being one of three important aging factors! And it isn't just about a positive impact on our biology/physiology, it is also key to weight loss, as water performs a crucial role in the fat-burning process (*Low-Fat Living*[8]).

Drink water to lose fat: "Water is the most significant anti-aging secret of all time."

(Bill Frank's Forever Young[45])

I will drink to that!

I HAVE SEEN THE ENEMY

The war is aging. To win the battles that we face, and ultimately the war, we need to identify what I call the major aging enemies, which one expert labels as aging accelerators. We also need to have a battle plan and the troops/weaponry needed to fight these enemies and win that war. The rest of this chapter will be dedicated to identifying those aging enemies and some general battle strategies to fight the fight. Chapter 3 and beyond will cover specific troops and weaponry we can use to win.

Here's how the aging accelerators shake out according to *Ten Years Younger*:[46]

1. Diet [i.e., glycation, which leads to AGEs].

2. Oxidative stress (which creates free radicals).

3. Inflammation.

4. Chronic stress.

5. Metabolic stress (imbalance between calories we consume and those we burn).

6. Physical inactivity.

7. Toxins (i.e., smoking, too much alcohol, pesticides, etc.).

Aging accelerators are clearly aging enemies. The three major aging enemies that we will consider first are: glycation, oxidation, and inflammation. We have already introduced the first two when we talked about skin (part 1, chapter 2, section 1). In this first section, we will discuss glycation and oxidation further. These are key foundational concepts to understand, as some of the other aging accelerators damage our body by producing AGEs and free radicals. In the next section, we will get into the third major aging enemy, chronic inflammation. Let's begin by talking about glycation because the effects of this enemy on aging are extensive and powerful!

Glycation: Sugar is sabotaging your health and making you age faster as sugar molecules attach themselves to proteins and fats = Advanced Glycation End-Products or, AGEs.

(The Immortality Edge[32])

It can't be said too often, either here or out in the communications world at large: ***sugar is really, really bad for us.*** For a *60 Minutes* story titled "Is Sugar Toxic" that CBS aired on April 1, 2012, Dr. Sanjay Gupta interviewed Dr. Robert Lusting, who called sugar toxic. I have read/heard other experts call it "poison."

Sugar is the basis for glycation, which occurs when sugar molecules we have ingested attach themselves to proteins and fats, as noted above, forming AGEs. You don't have to remember glycation, just remember that sugar leads to AGEs, and AGEs are a *major* aging enemy to how we *age*.

Numerous aging experts talk about the role of AGEs and how they age us. I had no idea before I did this research what they were or how impactful they are, and in fact, the term was unfamiliar to me (just another example of how much I learned from the aging authorities while writing this book). *Breaking the Aging Code*[68] states that no other molecule is as toxic to proteins as AGEs are. *Some of the harmful effects include eye damage, kidney damage, peripheral nerves and blood vessels damage; malfunction of the immune system; and failure of insulin to store glucose as energy with resulting muscle fatigue, high cholesterol, and added risk of heart attack and stroke.*[68] No question, this is a major aging enemy!

Anti-Aging Quick Tip: Avoid sugar to live longer with fewer wrinkles.

If that is not enough, as mentioned in part 1, wrinkles are a visible sign of AGEs because of the glucose (sugar) binding to protein (*Ageless Face, Ageless Mind*[21]). *The Immortality Edge*[32] describes what is seen as a whole range of physiologic effects and diseases related to AGEs:

- Accumulation of amyloid in the brain.

- Abnormal methylation (which is a body chemistry process that can lead to cervical cancer, colon cancer, heart disease, stroke, Alzheimer's and other bad conditions).

- Clumping of platelets.

- Damage to eyes.

Sugar we eat wreaks all kinds of aging havoc with our bodies! I'm thinking we might want to think twice before grabbing that cookie, or candy, or piece of pie, or…the list goes on and on. Remember, it is all about our choices. Enough said.

Anti-Aging Quick Tip: Use antioxidants from plants and spices to decelerate aging.

Now, let's focus on the second major bad guy in the aging process: oxidation, and its general internal impact on aging. We started this discussion when we talked about skin and skin care because free radicals created by sun radiation can damage skin. Oxygen is a paradox for us: it has life-giving energy, but if given the chance, it destroys the molecular components of the body just as surely as it rusts metal and burns buildings (*Freedom From Disease: How to Control Free Radicals, A Major Cause of Aging and Disease*[87]).

Oxygen is required for cell metabolism (chemical processes that are necessary for the maintenance of life), but in the process, free oxygen radicals are created. When these free radicals overwhelm the body's ability to remove them, oxidative stress can occur, causing cell and tissue damage. The free radicals are one electron short (highly unbalanced), so they steal electrons, which damages other molecules. They do this because they are driven to even up this imbalance, and this sends them in frenzied attacks against their molecular neighbors, becoming terrorists in our physical bodies.

Again from *Freedom From Disease*:[87] they can attack our DNA, which leads to dysfunction, mutation, and can even lead to cancer; they can attack enzymes and proteins, cell membranes (which in our blood vessels can lead to hardening of our arteries), and collagen (resulting in stiffness in the body). One aging authority lists the following free radical diseases:

Cancer, arteriosclerosis, atherosclerosis,
heart disease, strokes, emphysema,
maturity onset diabetes, rheumatoid
arthritis, ulcers, cataracts, Crohn's
disease, Behcet's disease, Reynaud's
disease, senility.[87]

Another aging expert states the following:

Free radicals contribute to at least fifty
major diseases, including atherosclerosis,
heart disease, rheumatoid arthritis, and lung
disease, as well as accelerated aging.

(Forever Young[71])

Free radicals are "a steady, significant onslaught against your body that intensifies with age" (*Prevention Positively Ageless*[4]). Like remembering AGEs are really bad, just remember that anything that creates free radicals is also really bad for aging. The good news is, we have great weaponry to fight these with both internal and external antioxidants, which act as "free radical scavengers," helping the body remove these damaging molecules and prevent and repair damage. These antioxidants play a lead role as an aging decelerator because they help prevent age-related diseases, they stimulate the immune system, they protect the nervous system and brain, and they prevent, or slow, the damage of aging (*Age Proof Your Body*[47]).

Anti-Aging Quick Tip: "Rustproof your cells with antioxidants." (*Bill Frank's Forever Young*[45])

Because we humans don't have built-in internal antioxidants, we need to acquire them in our diet (or in our skin-care products, for the external body), but what is cool is that the antioxidants that occur naturally in plants work in our bodies the same way they work for plants, as antioxidant shields (*The China Study*[75]). We will talk more about specific antioxidants as weapons in the next chapter, when we get to the foods we eat, including spices, a number of which are powerful antioxidants.

SECTION 2: THE FIRE WITHIN

"Smoldering inflammation" is the cause of most disease/aging because it produces

*an overabundance of damaging free
radicals in your system so you age faster,
you get sick, you die from disease.*

(Healthy, Sexy, Happy[28])

From the quote above, we see that the third major aging enemy, inflammation, creates free radicals. We know already from the last section that free radicals are a major aging enemy. *SuperHealth*[59] tells us that inflammation is an immune response to tissue that has been injured or irritated or has become diseased, and that when foreign irritants invade, inflammation rushes to the rescue to initiate the healing process. Our bodies use inflammation to repair damaged tissue and to kill pathogens, so it is a very important process, but as a double-edged sword, it also has negative effects,[59] including being one of the major risk factors for a heart attack.

This may sound familiar, since we have already learned that our cells need oxygen to create energy, but that process (oxidation) creates free radicals that are damaging; i.e., the oxygen paradox. Like oxygen, inflammation is both useful to our bodies and, unfortunately, sometimes hurtful. It can get out of hand, like too much inflammation in a joint and arthritis. Or, when is goes overboard, it is a precursor to most diseases, including cardiovascular disease (as mentioned above), stroke, cancer, diabetes,

Alzheimer's, macular degeneration, and cataracts, plus it plays a central role in speeding up physical aging.[59]

> **Anti-Aging Quick Tip: Here are some things that we want to avoid because they fuel inflammation: smoking, stress, chronic sleep deprivation, being overweight, lack of exercise, and diet. (*SuperHealth*[59])**

Gum disease is part of this "fire within" inflammation problem. It is an interesting, and very damaging, chronic inflammatory disease that begins as a bacterial infection that leads to inflammation. The chronic inflammation ends up destroying the gum and bone support around teeth, which results in 70 percent of all adult tooth loss. Chronic inflammatory gum disease contributes to diabetes (and diabetes contributes to gum disease), and it is linked to other serious diseases, including heart disease and stroke. A recent landmark study showed that gum disease treatment can lower annual medical costs for people with heart disease and stroke by almost three thousand dollars and one thousand dollars, respectively (website article[51]). This kind of intervention study was also done for gum disease and diabetes, and I think they demonstrate a very powerful connection.

In another report, some researchers speculated that the chronic inflammation of gum disease specifically may promote the growth of pancreatic cancer cells; that men with poor gum health had a 63 percent higher risk of developing pancreatic cancer, and high levels of a key gum disease bacteria was linked to a greater risk of dying of pancreatic and colorectal cancer (website article[41]). The American Academy of Periodontology, in its e-news *This Week in Perio*, also reported that a growing number of studies suggest a role for infections (primarily of the stomach and gums) in pancreatic cancer. That same issue reported that bacteria linked to gum disease traveled to the brains of people with Alzheimer's disease, suggesting that dental hygiene plays a role in the development of the memory-robbing illness (website article[59]).

> **Anti-Aging Quick Tip: DON'T avoid flossing to avoid chronic inflammation in your gum tissue.**

So, you don't have to remember any of the aforementioned details, do remember that chronic inflammation is a major aging enemy and that "floss for life" may be a very good motto for longevity.

STRESSED OUT: AN ENEMY INTERPLAY

Aging accelerators can also interact with each other, joining destructive forces, creating even more potent threats. I would remind the reader here of a favorite quote from Oscar Wilde that I mentioned in the prologue and have used in my lectures for almost thirty years: "The truth is rarely pure, and never simple." This applies perfectly to the three major aging enemies, because they are not entirely distinct and they often work in conjunction with each other, or fuel each other, creating a complex process of aging poorly.

It turns out that there is, in fact, a lot of interplay among the major aging accelerators, and an example of that is chronic stress. As noted earlier in this section (and in chapter 1 when we talked about stress damaging our brains), stress fuels chronic inflammation, so this is an example of the interplay of aging enemies because we know that chronic inflammation produces free radicals, which are a major aging enemy. Another double-edge sword, another paradox: stress can be good, but it can also be bad for us. Good stress can be very motivating, even inspiring.

But bad chronic stress can do a lot of damage! Chronic stress accelerates the aging process (*Transcend: Nine Steps to Living Well Forever*[9]), including killing brain cells, and contributing to Alzheimer's disease, as we talked about in the preceding chapter (*Beautiful Brain, Beautiful You*[11]). Can we compare stress to smoking? Well, consider this: a very interesting study in the *American Journal of Cardiology* online (September 12, 2012) concluded: "Taken together, the studies found that people who felt stressed were 27 percent more likely later to be diagnosed with coronary heart disease, be hospitalized with the condition, or die from it" (website article[50]). One of the authors, Donald Edmondson, said the rise in heart disease risk related to stress is equivalent to smoking five cigarettes a day.

In addition to direct damage from chronic inflammation and the free radicals it produces, stress can also handcuff our stem cells, weakening their ability to repair age-related damage (*You Staying Young: The Owner's Manual for Extending Your Warranty*[5]), plus undermining our immune system (*The Longevity Bible*[42]).

Anti-Aging Quick Tip: Play in the dirt a little to help win the aging battle.

Speaking of the immune system (one of the three most important factors that affect aging), I think we don't play in the dirt enough anymore! Mud pies were great fun, and I believe good for the development of our immune system the way it was intended to be developed. Think about our HG (hunter-gatherer) ancestors—we need their lifestyle of outdoor exposure! I believe we have gotten too clean, too sterile, too protective, and even too housebound in a lot of instances. Dig in the dirt. Get off that keyboard or smart phone and go outside to play. Gee whiz, do something!

As anecdotal evidence, when I was still in clinical practice, I saw a lot of people each day but never got a cold or the flu. Now that I have quit practicing, I get many of the colds and flu that come around. This makes a lot of biologic sense to me. I seriously need to get out more and shake a few hands so that I develop protection toward what's out there! I could consider politics, since I am jobless, but who can put up with that stuff? So, I think I will just keep playing in the dirt and try to get out more...

Moving on from that aside (we will come back to the immune system soon), stress also can contribute to GI problems, type 2 diabetes, cancer, rheumatoid arthritis, heart disease, and stroke, plus anxiety, depression, difficulty concentrating, insomnia, and substance abuse such as compulsive eating, gambling, drinking, or sexual activity (*Transcend: Nine Steps to Living Well Forever*[9]). Further, it increases fat deposited in the abdomen by increasing cortisol and insulin (*Low-Fat Living*[8]). It is common knowledge that belly fat is really bad for us, and in the 160-plus written works I looked at, this was verified over and over again.

We already know that fat fuels inflammation, creating damaging free radicals. We also know that sleep deprivation leads to inflammation, as do a poor diet, lack of exercise, and being overweight, which we will talk more about next. I think you can see the interplay I am talking about. Think about the word disease. I hear another mother's voice: as my mother-in-law used to say, dissect the word and it says dis-ease. Discomfort, uneasiness: stress creates these kinds of feelings, leading potentially to all kinds of physical and emotional issues (more about this, and ideas to help deal with it, in part 3).

WEIGHT: AN ENEMY INTERPLAY

Another example of enemy interplay is when we are overweight. This is called metabolic stress (or weight loss stress), which is the imbalance between calories we consume and calories burned, according to *Ten Years Younger*.[46] If we are overweight and unhealthy, we have the **enemy free radicals** in our system that are damaging to mitochondria and DNA; our body and brain are breaking down on a cellular level more than they are rebuilding; we're suffering from insulin resistance (a condition which, as we noted earlier, is where insulin becomes less effective at lowering blood sugar, which results in increased blood sugar, which can cause adverse health effects); we have smoldering inflammation (fat cells trigger inflammation) in our tissues (especially brain); and we're exhausted because mitochondria are generating less energy (*Healthy, Sexy, Happy*[28]). The damaged DNA can lead to the initiation of certain cancers (*Forever Young*[71]). In addition, a just-published literature review reported that there is an association between gum disease and obesity and this association is chronic inflammation (website article[53]), which we know is an aging accelerator.

A recent study (of mice), quoted in the e-newsletter *Food for the Brain* (website article[21]), illustrated a direct link between a high-fat diet and obesity and their contribution to the development of Alzheimer's disease. This is seriously heavy stuff. What is great is that in today's world, we know a lot about it and we are discovering ways to prevent/reduce/reverse aging poorly. I think we all want to age as well as possible, and I can't think of any person wanting to suffer, or watch someone else suffer, the horrible torturing life of Alzheimer's. The literal and figurative weight of this cannot be ignored. Enough said about that.

THE SUGAR FLOOD AND DEVASTATION

Another example of enemy interplay is more bad news about a real bad actor in the aging process, sugar. As we have already established, sugar is another true, major enemy of aging, period; it is simply plain, non-sugarcoated bad for us. The interplay of the three major aging factors continues here, since in addition to inflammation creating free radicals, sugar (which creates AGEs, and, as discussed earlier, are very damaging on their own) can lead to chronic elevated blood sugar, contributing to inflammation, which can also inflict significant damage by releasing free radicals. Aha! All three of the major aging enemies have converged in one place, related to—sadly, yes—sugar.

> Bathing cells in sugar produces an inflammatory state. Chronic elevated blood sugar triggers elevated insulin levels, which is pro-inflammatory [contributes to chronic inflammation].
>
> (Breaking the Aging Code[68])

From *Healthy, Sexy, Happy*:[28] The goal of eating and living in a healthy, youthful way is to keep insulin levels balanced; if we eat too much sugar, insulin is released to store sugar into cells; at some point, if we keep flooding our bloodstream with sugar, cells will be filled to capacity so they can't take in more sugar; receptors are shut down for insulin (i.e., insulin resistance), which leads the pancreas to pump out more insulin, putting too much in the blood (which is pro-inflammatory, as noted above). The body then has to turn extra sugar into fat, stowed away around our waist first and leading to, again, chronic inflammation and free radicals. Eventually even fat cells will be stuffed, leading to high blood sugar (type 2 diabetes).[28] The aging enemies can really gang up on us if we are not watchful and careful!

DISEASE INTERPLAY

The last interplay I want to touch on before we go on to discuss the other aging accelerators is disease interplay and the aging enemies. An example of disease interplay is that diabetes can cause and be caused by chronic inflammation, according to *Breaking the Aging Code*.[68] So can atherosclerosis, heart valve dysfunction, obesity, congestive heart failure, and some digestive system diseases.[68] As has already been noted, gum disease, a chronic inflammatory disease, can exacerbate out-of-control blood sugar and diabetes can accelerate gum disease. This is the most well-understood link between gum disease and the serious, systemic diseases. I think you can see that aging does not happen in isolation. It happens as a cocktail of aging accelerators and factors coupled with our bodies' abilities to handle and respond to them. This is why this subject is complex, with many factors/players, and why it has to be fought with a toolbox full of aging tidbits to decrease the impact of the aging enemies.

SECTION 3: HEAR THE BATTLE CRY

So, we have reviewed five of the seven major aging accelerators. The sixth, toxins, will come in the next chapter, and physical inactivity/activity will be covered in total in chapter 5. Temporarily, I would like to leave off identifying the enemies and turn to talking about some of the general battle strategies to fight the ones we have identified so far. What are the foundational principles that we can use to fight back? From *SuperHealth*,[59] there are six general big-picture strategies, combined with steps we can take to fight cancer, control heart disease, reverse aging, shrink our waistline, and be our vital best:

1. **Control your genes (nutrigenomics) through omega-3 fatty acids and resveratrol (i.e., you can turn on "good" genes and turn off "bad" genes).**

2. Become an environmentalist and detoxify your body; i.e., avoid pesticides, industrial waste, and eat "green" with soy, apples, tea, onions, cruciferous veggies, garlic, and spices that help reduce the harmful effects of those toxins that do slip in.

3. Watch your waistline, burn those calories.

4. Control inflammation; i.e., avoid sugar, avoid smoking, decrease stress, get enough sleep, avoid being overweight, get exercise, and include superfoods in your diet [and, do not avoid flossing].

5. Keep up appearances; i.e., there is a definite correlation between how your skin ages and the foods you eat.

6. Preserve your senses; i.e., flame out at the finish line still being able to see, hear, smell, taste, feel, and think your way independently in the world.

We have touched on several of these general strategies. We know that we need to reduce our sugar intake as much as possible to decrease AGEs and chronic inflammation. We also know that we have to fight free radicals and overboard inflammation, so we need to develop some antioxidant and anti-inflammatory protective warriors to help us fight those bad guys. The entire next chapter will share specific warriors in what we eat (i.e., things like eating foods high in antioxidants, anti-AGE foods, anti-inflammatory foods, and taking in phytonutrients, which are plant compounds thought to promote health and prevent disease).

We also have already talked about aging skin issues, the senses, and some of the issues of being overweight. We will talk about dealing with toxins at the end of section 1 in the next chapter, and the role of burning calories with exercise in chapter 5. As far as nutrigenomics goes, I came across only a couple of the aging authorities who talked on this concept, but there is evidence that we can control our gene expression in a good way, by turning on "good" genes and turning off "bad" genes.[59,71] We will talk about this a little more when we discuss the "free radical fighters" in the next chapter.

Another anti-aging strategy that I introduced early in this chapter and would add to the *SuperHealth*[59] strategy list is to bolster our immune system, which are our internal protective troops against invaders. As we have said before, *RealAge*[26] identifies the immune system as one of the three most important factors that affect aging. Anything we can do that has a positive influence on this system helps us win the aging battle, so it is worth our time to identify those strategies. We covered some of them earlier. In addition, WebMD (website article[42]) offers the following suggestions to strengthen the immune system: reduce your stress; enjoy regular sex; get a pet; build a strong social network; keep a positive attitude; have a laugh; eat your antioxidants; take your vitamins if your diet is lacking; avoid empty calories such as those in fast foods, snack foods, candy, and soda; consider herbs and supplements; exercise; sleep well; limit alcohol; stop smoking; and wash your hands. Do you see now how everything is connected, interwoven, intertwined?

According to a *Newsmax* article (website article[43]), boosting your immune system may be more important than vaccines (such as that for shingles), which may contain brain-toxic additives and may be contaminated with organisms. When I talked about stress, I mentioned that I thought we should play in the dirt more to bolster our immune system. Apparently, the book *You Staying Young*[5] agrees with that idea, among a few others:

BATTLE OF THE INVADERS

❏ Singing and laughing are good for the immune system.

❏ Exposure to "dirt" can strengthen your immunity.

❏ As can relaxation techniques, so meditate daily.

☐ Omega-3 boosts immunity by getting omega-6/ omega-3 at their best ratio.

I love this list, and I think the reader would agree that these are pretty easy to incorporate into our lifestyles with very little price to be paid, literally or figuratively. That is great ROI. Yahoo!

CHAPTER 3:

FUELS TO FEED THE FLAME

SECTION 1: THE BATTLE PLAN

News flash: studies have found that diet and exercise can slow aging not only at the general, somatic (body) level, but at the cellular level of the telomeres (which are the ends of our chromosomes that carry our genetic information). These telomeres shorten with age, making us more vulnerable to disease, so these healthy diet and exercise habits can slow aging at levels from our whole body to our cells (website article[23]). In this chapter and the next, we will look at these two important graceful aging strategies with all their age-improving effects.

A FIGHT TO THE END

We are literally and figuratively in the fight of our lives against the aging enemies—fighting to live long, look great, and, most importantly, be healthy. The goal is to win the battle, and to do that, we need warriors, their weapons, and a battle plan that capitalizes on their potential impact. We defined the major enemies in the previous chapter, and at the end we shared one authoritative view of some general, big-picture strategies for that fight against those major aging enemies. This chapter will get into more specific strategies related to how we can eat in a more positive aging way by identifying the food warriors and their weapons, ending with some diet plan strategies that utilize them in the battle to help us achieve our goal of youthful, long, healthy lives. The awesome news is, there are lots of foods and spices to choose from that are excellent troops for this battle.

There are two prongs to this fight. One is to identify the warrior troops and their weaponry that will serve us in our quest to win. The other is to figure out how to change our current diet to incorporate the good guys, all the while getting rid of the unhealthy aging bad guys. For many, like me, this requires some significant change in the way we shop, design meals, cook, and eat, including *when* we eat.

> **Anti-Aging Quick Tip:** A Harvard study showed that men who skipped breakfast had a 27 percent increased risk for heart attack or death from heart disease compared to men who started their day with a healthy meal. (website article[58])

Change is never easy, but I have proven to myself that this works by seeing an improved fasting blood sugar score as well as a significantly reduced "bad" cholesterol score and improved blood pressure readings at my last physical, not to mention a RealAge biologic age that is just shy of eight years younger than my chronologic age—all without taking any medications!

What I did to help make the process easier was that I made the changes in baby steps. Initially I focused on eating more of the "good" foods that I already liked and wasn't eating much, while I started working on not eating the "bad" foods that I was kind of neutral about. I gradually added some new "good for me" foods that I had doubts about, like spaghetti squash and sweet potatoes, and let go of or minimized some foods that I liked but weren't that great for my well-being.

As part of this process, I also started experimenting with spices that I had never used, chief among those being turmeric, and increasing the amount of some that I already used, like cinnamon. The other very important thing that I am still using to help me with these big changes comes from *The Paleo Solution*.[15] An 80 percent effort to eat right produces 95 percent of the benefit offered, so I still eat foods that are not on the "eat healthy, age well" list, but I see that as part of the whole process and being perfectly imperfectly human, not as a sign of failure.

ROLL CALL: THE TROOPS

Because there is lots of authoritative information in this area, I am going to approach the subject by subdividing it into some bite-sized (excuse the pun) chunks. These chunks are my way of sorting and organizing the information so that it is more digestible (the puns are free-flowing in this subject matter!). My list of the warrior categories is as follows:

1. *Those that fight free radicals with their antioxidant weapons.*

2. *The anti-AGE foods with their weapons to control blood sugar and insulin levels.*

3. *The anti-inflammatory troops with their inherent weaponry.*

4. *The health promoting and disease preventing troops with their phytonutrient weapons.*

5. *The troops that enhance detoxification.*

I have chosen to look at the spice weaponry separately in section 2, as they are powerful crossover weaponry that are antioxidant, fight AGEs, AND are phytonutrient (more on this shortly). In the third section of this chapter, we will look at approaches that group foods into diet battle plan troops. In that same section, we will also look at infiltrator foods that may be in our current battle plan but need to be put into detention, on the "not to eat or eat minimally" list. Section 4 has a few last tidbits on the dining experience itself.

FREE RADICAL FIGHTERS

As we talked about in the previous chapter, free radicals are said to contribute to at least fifty major diseases PLUS accelerated aging. They are truly one of the very damaging aging enemies worth fighting!

Free radicals are a steady, significant onslaught against your body that intensifies with age.

(Prevention Positively Ageless[4])

So, how do we deal with THIS enemy in particular? The key is to strike a balance between the number of free radicals generated and the body's defense and repair systems (*Freedom from Disease*[87]). One strategy in the battle plan to fight free radicals internally is to intake potent warriors via the foods we choose to eat (versus skin, where we actually apply them topically). These warriors are known as antioxidants. These ready-made, and nature-made, molecules sacrifice by donating electrons to "capture" free radicals[87]—thus my label, the free radical fighters.

An example of how important these antioxidants are is illustrated here. One of the very scary things to worry about, and something I think many boomers do worry about, is Alzheimer's disease. A very good website, FoodForTheBrain.org (website link[8]), had an article about the prevention of this awful disease. On their list of ways to prevent this debilitating and deadly illness are a couple related to what we eat. One prevention strategy that the article mentions is to stay away from sugar and refined foods. This should sound oh so very familiar to us; we paid attention to and gave recognition to this concept in chapter 2 on more than one occasion.

Another strategy they suggest is to increase your intake of antioxidants (website article[8]). Let's say that again: by increasing free radical fighter antioxidants in our diet, we can help prevent Alzheimer's. Wow! These antioxidant fighters are clearly warriors we want to take advantage of. A logical question is, can we get those antioxidants in our vitamins and supplements?

When I think about it, what makes biologic sense echoes the aging authority in *Prevention Positively Ageless*[4] who said that antioxidants are neutralizing, but antioxidants from a bottle can actually have "pro-aging, pro-oxidizing" effects. Perhaps the man-made chemical concoction in that plastic bottle cannot compare to what nature provides? This, to me, is not only conceivable, but biologically sound.

WebMD also reports that it is best to get vitamins, minerals, and antioxidants by eating them, rather than taking a pill (website article[55]). There seems to be an inexplicable synergy between our somas and Mother Nature's antioxidants found naturally in food. From *1001 Ways to Stay Young*:[39] eating food as close to its natural state as possible helps ensure maximum exposure to youth-enhancing nutrients.

But of course, like prescription medicines, vitamins and/or supplements are sometimes still needed. For example, I am, and have been since birth, lactose intolerant, which makes it difficult for me to get all the calcium I need. So, I take a calcium supplement most days. For a long while, I also took vitamin C, Centrum Silver, and vitamin D every day on the recommendation of my internist, but since my very positive diet changes over the last couple of years, I do not take C any longer, as I eat lots of fruit and vegetables, and I take the others infrequently, when I feel like what I am eating has been deficient, falling in that 20 percent "not so healthy" category. My bottom line is that I recommend, and prefer myself, natural whenever possible! The *New Longevity Diet*[61] talks about this:

- ❐ "The answer lies not in unnatural, manmade sources, but in the foods we love."
- ❐ "Longevity nutrients are ready, willing and able to prevent aging."
- ❐ "So instead of looking for some new drug or chemical to retard aging, look to nature."
- ❐ The idea: Eat the right amount of wholesome, tasty foods to boost our immune system, digestion, respiration, nervous system, reproductive system, circulatory system, endocrine system,

musculo-skeletal system, and skin systems so that it all runs like well-oiled machinery.

To take this concept further, I am completely convinced, due to all the book research and my science background, that Mother Nature supplies us with everything we need to be healthy and live long. We don't need to pore over the drugstore or specialty store shelves looking for the magic pill. We don't need more laboratory concoctions that are promoted as "the answer." What we need is to study very intently what is provided naturally, and there, I believe, we will find the solutions to our aging and disease issues. From algae or seaweed in the ocean to acai berries from Central and South America, I believe that the answers to all our questions and concerns are already here. It is not required for the reader to agree with me, but maybe at least consider it *food* for thought.

Nature is doing her best each moment to make us well. She exists for no other end. With the least inclination to be well, we should not be sick.

—Henry David Thoreau

So, let's talk some specifics. *Prevention Positively Ageless*,[4] along with many of the aging authorities I reviewed, provides us some ideas on what these anti-aging weapons are: blueberries, mushrooms, veggies, cocoa, red wine, green tea, coffee, and olive oil (which is also heart healthy and may help prevent cancer) can swoop in to halt free radicals; sweeteners with antioxidants include agave nectar, honey, and molasses. As an aside about mushrooms, *Forever Young*[71] tells us that throughout Asia, certain mushrooms have played important roles in maintaining health, preserving youth, and increasing longevity. Being a big mushroom lover, this is more great news for me. This same aging expert also tells us about a powerful, natural, combined antioxidant/anti-inflammatory carotenoid that I had not ever heard called by name:

Astaxanthin (a carotenoid) is one of the most powerful of all-natural antioxidants. Found in seafood, giving pink and red to salmon, shrimp and lobster. Its significant anti-inflammatory power is vital to the maintenance of youthful vitality.

Anti-Aging Quick Tip: Eat salmon and drink red wine to switch on protective genes.

An interesting tidbit that I uncovered in my research on aging (SuperHealth[59]) is that some of these antioxidants, like resveratrol [found in red and purple grapes, along with red wine] and omega-3 fatty acids [in foods such as salmon, walnuts, soybeans, certain oils, winter squash, etc.] can change gene expression. *Forever Young*[71] states it as such: with diet you can switch on protective genes and switch off genes that may have a negative effect on your health. This is called nutrigenomics, which we mentioned in the previous chapter.

Salmon is also probably the world's most heart-healthy source of protein. Omega-3 fatty acids protect heart health, inhibit inflammation, act as natural antidepressants, increase feelings of well-being, and help keep skin young, supple and radiant.

(Forever Young[71]*)*

Boy, salmon is right up there at the top with its anti-aging power. I try to eat salmon once each week, my favorite preparation being poached with a little low-fat organic chicken stock or white wine and a dry rub of favorite spices, or coated with a "pesto" of olive oil and fresh garden herbs (savory, thyme, and garlic, for instance). Sounds good even at this moment, it being only 10:00 a.m. and I have already eaten breakfast! Once again, I am so fortunate to live up here in the Pacific Northwest with our excellent access to this amazing fish.

ANTI-AGE WARRIORS

Another strategy in our battle plan is to fight the AGEs enemy. We know that AGEs are very toxic and very aging. As we learned in chapter 2, they can damage eyes, kidneys, blood vessels, and our immune system. From *Ageless Face, Ageless Mind*,[21] we get tidbits on how to fight THESE bad guys:

AGE Stop

- To keep the body healthy, and the skin youthful and radiant, we want

> an anti-AGE diet that is designed to control blood sugar and insulin levels.
> * Avoid sugar and high-sugar foods, MSG, salt, preservatives, processed foods, food coloring, high-fructose corn syrup, pasta, breads, pastry, baked goods, and snack foods.
> * Choose made by nature, not in the lab.
> * Do not cook on high heat or for prolonged periods (creates AGEs).

Basically, we want to avoid SAD, which is the acronym for the Standard American Diet, an unfortunately sad alternative to healthy eating. And to make matters worse, in my view, we have taken this "sad" SAD to many/most parts of the rest of the world! It is embarrassing to think that we are making others in the world sick and obese like we are. I will get off this soapbox right now, as it is enough said, and others say it much better than I.

INFLAMMATORY FIGHTERS

A third aging gracefully strategy is to fight the aging enemy inflammation. Something that may be of interest comes from the article titled "The Latest Science on Aging." It was reported that those who drank one daily alcoholic beverage during middle age were more likely to grow old without developing any physical or mental limitations, or chronic diseases, maybe because moderate drinking can reduce inflammation, raise HDL (good) cholesterol, and improve insulin function (*O Magazine*[89]).

I personally grew up with the idea that alcohol is a very bad thing, but as I have matured in age and experience, I have realized that alcohol problems, like many/most/all our problems, are really about anything in excess. As Aristotle advised, all things in moderation. I appreciate now that alcohol can make a positive contribution to our aging process, which goes to show you the value of research and how it most certainly provides more food (or in this case, drink) for thought.

There are other authoritative tidbits on battling inflammation. *The Anti-Aging Fitness Prescription*[63] tells us to:

☐ Eat more omega-3 fatty acid rich foods (walnuts, flaxseed, cold-water fish like salmon, sardines, trout).

☐ Eat more food rich in vitamin C (strawberries, oranges, red peppers).

☐ Eat more foods rich in vitamin E (nuts, veggie-based oils).

☐ Eat less saturated fat.

☐ Reduce body fat.

☐ Exercise regularly.

☐ Don't smoke.

Finally, noteworthy, and to me somewhat surprising, pineapple has a broad range of interesting properties, including its natural anti-inflammatory weapon, bromelain.

• Pineapple is high in manganese, a mineral that is critical to development of strong bones and connective tissue. A cup of fresh pineapple will give you nearly 75% of the recommended daily amount.

- Bromelain, a proteolytic enzyme, is the key to pineapple's value. Proteolytic means "breaks down protein," which is why pineapple is known to be a digestive aid. It helps the body digest proteins more efficiently.

- Bromelain is also considered an effective anti-inflammatory. Regular ingestion of at least one-half cup of fresh pineapple daily is purported to relieve painful joints common to osteoarthritis. It produces mild pain relief.

- Fresh pineapple is not only high in this vitamin [C], but because of the bromelain, it has the ability to reduce mucus in the throat. If you have a cold with a productive cough, add pineapple to your diet. Those individuals who eat fresh pineapple daily report fewer sinus problems related to allergies.

- Pineapple is also known to discourage blood clot development. This makes it a valuable dietary addition for frequent fliers and others who may be at risk for blood clots.

(website article[14])

HEALTH PROMOTING AND DISEASE PREVENTION TROOPS

Another troop of excellent warriors in the healthy longevity, anti-aging battle are called phytonutrients. These weapons are highly nutritious plant compounds that promote health and prevent disease. They work because plants produce these substances to protect themselves from bacteria and viruses (website article[63]). Superfoods is a term sometimes used to describe foods with high phytonutrient content (along with salmon with its omega-3 oil). Some examples:

Superfoods: wild salmon, blueberries, broccoli, tomatoes, soy, flaxseed, oats, strawberries.

(The 100 Year Lifestyle[31])

One aging authority shared this tidbit that I would have never thought about, or guessed, might be important:

Watercress is an extraordinary superfood with cancer protection and it is a powerful antioxidant.

(Forever Young[71])

The following table, provided in a website article, identifies the health promoting and disease fighting phytonutrient troops and their specific weaponry.

FOOD	PHYTONUTRIENTS	BENEFITS
Berries (blueberries, raspberries, blackberries, strawberries, etc.)	Anthocyanidins, Ellagic Acid	Both have antioxidant activity which may aid in prevention of certain cancers. Anthocyanidins may also help prevent heart disease. Berries are rich in vitamin C, another antioxidant and soluble fiber which can help lower cholesterol. Studies are also showing that blueberries may aid in weight loss .
Chili Peppers (hot peppers, any variety)	Capsaicin	Giving chilis their heat, capsaicin may also aid in weight loss by boosting metabolism and stimulating the release of endorphins ("feel-good" hormones). It may also interfere with the growth of cancer cells and prevent blood clotting. Chilis are also high in vitamin C.

 Citrus Fruit (oranges, grapefruit, lemons, etc.	Flavanones, Flavonoids, Coumarins, D-limonene, Carotenoids	D-limonene, found in citrus skin neutralizes cancer promoting toxins. Carotenoids not only protect the eyes from free radical damage or cancer. Flavonoids act as antioxidants and help lower cholesterol. High in vitamin C and pectin which can help with weight loss, hence the grapefruit diet and the popularity of the juice diet. Lastly, the powerful combination of phytochemicals in citrus can actually protect the phytochemicals of other foods so to be utilized by the body. A great example is the catechins in green tea (which can aid in weight loss): Adding lemon protects the potency of the catechins.

|

Cruciferous Vegetables (cauliflower, broccoli, brussels sprouts, cabbage) | Indoles, Isothiocyanates, Carotenoids | Isothiocyanates, particularly Sulforaphane, found in cruciferous vegetables can help neutralize cancer causing toxins thus preventing damage to cells. They may also interfere with tumor growth. Indoles may reduce the risk of breast cancer by making estrogen less potent. Carotenoids prevent free radical damage to the eyes and may also reduce the risk of certain cancers. Besides being high in fiber and low in calories, cruciferous vegetables are also included in many popular detox diets for weight loss, and the alkaline soup diet. |

	Lignans	Lignans are a phyto-chemical that also act as a phytoestrogen, which means they weakly mimic the effects of estrogen in the body. Though research is still going on as to lignans' potential benefits and side effects (especially in men), one recent study found that diets high in lignans are associated with <u>healthier weights and blood sugar levels in postmenopausal women</u>.
Flax Seeds and Flax Flour		
Onions, Garlic, Shallots, Leeks, Scallions	Allylic sulfides, Flavonoids	Allylic sulfides and flavo-noids may aid in neu-tralizing cancer-causing toxins and free radicals, and have been associ-ated with lowering risks of colon and stomach cancers.

Herbs and Spices (thyme, rosemary, basil, ginger, turmeric, etc.)	Carnaso, Phenols, Terpenoids, Gingerols, Curcumin, etc.	Fresh herbs and spices are loaded with antioxidants and phytochemicals which can help prevent the growth of tumor cells and aid in neutralizing free radicals. Curcumin, the active phytochemical in turmeric (used in curry and also gives mustard its coloring) has shown strong potential in <u>preventing the growth of fat cells</u>, as well as preventing <u>Alzheimer's and heart disease</u>.
Legumes (black beans, kidney beans, lentils, etc.)	Isoflavonoids, Lignans, Phytic acid, Phytosterols, Saponins	High in fiber and protein, legumes are a great addition to any healthy weight loss diet. Insoluble fiber and phytosterols naturally lower cholesterol levels, while flavonoids lower risks of cancer and heart disease.
Nuts	Ellagic Acid, Saponins	Along with nuts' high content of healthy unsaturated fats, ellagic acid and saponins may also help protect the heart and blood vessels.

Yellow and Orange Fruits and Vegetables; Dark Leafy Greens	Carotenoids (especially beta-carotene, lutein, and zeaxanthin)	Carotenoids are well-known for protecting the eyes from free radical damage, but they may also aid in the prevention of cancers and in strengthening the immune system.
Red Wine and Grapes (red or purple)	Flavonols, Resveratrol, Anthocyanidins, Ellagic Acid	Resveratrol is a phyto-chemical that has become a popular weight loss and antiaging supplement. It may reduce the risk of cancer by preventing free radical damage. Anthocyanidins and ellagic acid also act as antioxidants. Flavonols, especially quercitin in grapes may also help protect the heart.

Soy and Soy Products (tofu, soymilk)	Isoflavonoids (genistein and daidzein), Lignans, Phytosterols, Saponins	High in complete protein and low in calories soy is a great diet food, especially for women as the isoflavonoids and lignans may help prevent certain cancers, particularly breast cancer. Lignans are also associated with healthier body weights and blood sugar levels in postmenopausal women. Phytosterols and saponins may also help prevent cancer.
Dark Chocolate, Green and Black Tea	Flavonols (especially catechins and EGCG – epigallocatechin-3-gallate), Flavonoids	EGCG has potent anti-cancer effects and helps protect the heart and arteries. Catechins act as antioxidants and have been associated with weight loss. A recent study found that catechins can help reduce abdominal fat by enhancing the effects of exercise. While green tea is well-known for its benefits, the phytochemicals in black tea also have potent health benefits, including controlling blood sugar levels.

Tomatoes	Carotenoids (especially Lycopene)	A potent antioxidant, lycopene may reduce the risk of certain cancers, while protecting the heart, vessels, and eyes from free radical damage.
Grains (whole, minimally processed such as wheat, oats, brown rice, barley, etc.)	Saponins, Terpenoids, Phytic acid, Ellagic acid	Saponins may help prevent colon cancer by neutralizing free radicals and toxins in the intestines. Terpenoids, phytic acid, and ellagic acid may also neutralize the effects of free radicals, and reduce the risks for heart disease and cancer. Whole grains are rich in fiber, vitamins, and phytonutrients, which are all helpful as part of a healthy weight loss diet. Refined grains have had most of the fiber and nutrients stripped away. Enriched grains have been heavily processed with basic vitamins added; the phytonutrients/chemicals are impossible to replace.

(website article[15])

I am in awe, and am getting hungry merely sharing what we have covered so far, but we are not done yet. From the preceding extensive chart, I think you can appreciate the variety that we have available to us in the form of great foods and spices that are wonderfully good for us. Choose the ones that call you at first glance, and then relook at the chart in a month or two to possibly add others to your list. As we have noted before, how we age is all about the choices we make every day, including what we choose by hand to mouth. I like an analogy that Sanjay Gupta used when he was interviewed about his book, *Chasing Life*[95]: "Living well now is like putting money in a savings account. The dividends will come later, as you age. The better you are at "saving," the richer you will be when it comes time to reap the rewards." Like saving money for retirement, starting young leads to greater riches, so it is never too early, and most definitely never too late, in life to make good choices for ourselves.

ATTENTION, DETOX TROOPS

The last anti-aging warrior I want to touch on is the group of foods that have detoxification effects. Again, the list is long with lots of potential, so "choose your weapons" and add to that savings account!

Garlic is the single most important cleansing, detoxifying, and blood-purifying herb we have.

(Gary Null's Power Aging[77])

I think I must have been Italian in a former life, as I love all things Italian. Having always been a garlic and onion lover, I think of including both in many things I cook. Needless to say, I was thrilled to have them both validated in my research as being great for our bodies. Something else I was excited about: cilantro is a chelator of heavy metals (*Transcend: Nine Steps to Living Well Forever*[9]). I love cilantro, both fresh and in a lot of things! There are a number of other detox warriors, including those on this list from *Your Skin, Younger.*[69]

Other Detox Troops

Brassica family veggies support growth of beneficial bacteria in the gut and have been shown to enhance cellular detoxification:

- *Arugula*
- *Bok choy*
- *Broccoli*
- *Broccoli sprouts*
- *Broccolini*
- *Brussels sprouts*
- *Cabbage*
- *Cauliflower*
- *Chinese broccoli*
- *Daikon (white radish)*
- *Horseradish*
- *Kale*
- *Kohlrabi [a stout cultivar of cabbage]*
- *Mustard greens*
- *Watercress*

These same vegetables (also called cruciferous) have been identified as foods to **enhance elimination of cancer-causing compounds** from your system, along with turmeric, garlic, rosemary, and soy (*Ten Years Younger*[46]). Let's focus in on this for a moment: we can choose to eat certain things that not only taste great but may enhance the elimination of cancer-causing compounds in our bodies. *Cha-ching, cha-ching.* THAT is powerful stuff. I hear the mother's voice again: the old maternal adage that veggies are good for us is spot-on!

SECTION 2: SPICE IT UP COOKING LIVENED UP

Hey, those Spice Girls may have been onto something—spicing it up is really, truly good for us! It seems spices have almost thirty different nutrients in them, according to *Younger (Thinner) You Diet*.[33] I find that cooking with more spices not only livens up my mouth and the food I put in it, but it livens up the cooking experience with wonderfully enticing aromas and bright colors! I hope you will enjoy the information provided here and will use it to bring new meaning to that "spice it up" phrase!

I wasn't using spices nearly as much before the research for this book as I am now, and I have renewed a love of the smells and colors of spices. One that I mention throughout the book is turmeric, which I have truly fallen for, especially on baked sweet potatoes or chicken breast chunks browned in olive oil and garlic—good, good stuff. Turmeric is the anti-aging, anti-oxidant, anti-inflammatory, and anti-cancer super spice. It has a wonderful saffron color and an almost nutty taste that I have really grown to love. It is included on the list of anti-aging spices, along with others, from *1001 Ways to Stay Young Naturally*,[39] those being turmeric, curcumin, ginger, garlic, and onion.

> The single most promising food-derived compound to combat cancer, based on the current body of scientific evidence, is the curcuminoids found in turmeric.
>
> (Forever Young[71])

1001 Ways to Stay Young Naturally also reports that turmeric and green tea seem to enhance each other's health-giving properties. A recent *Prime Time News* report (website article[56]) and Dr. Sanjay Gupta, in his book *Chasing Life*,[95] talk about a supplement being studied that reverses cell aging in genes and that has, as partial ingredients, both green tea and turmeric. Initial findings indicate the supplement may be very effective at combating oxidative stress and free radicals. It seems that a convergence of expert opinion is occurring that validates this information for me because, as I have said before, when experts disagree on something, none of them probably have the answer exactly right, but when a number of experts coming from differing vantage points do agree, I have found those to be valid truisms. Take a good look at green tea and turmeric to include in the aging gracefully pathway. These are very exciting times where aging is concerned!

Another very powerful spice that I have always loved to use is cinnamon. It reduces blood sugar levels, reduces AGEs, is antibacterial and antifungal, and the scent enhances cognitive processing, including attention, memory, and visual-motor speed (*Ageless Face, Ageless Mind*[21]). It is also a powerful antioxidant and, according to *Forever* Young,[71] it may help treat melanoma. What tablet from a plastic bottle can beat that and taste so good? I think none.

> **Anti-Aging Quick "Hot" Tip: Find some capsaicin to liven up your diet and help burn fat.**

For those of us who want to boost our metabolism, burn more fat, and lose weight faster, we want to eat more hot pepper spices, which have capsaicin in them. Lucky me again: I LOVE jalapenos, Serrano peppers, red pepper flakes, etc., so this is great news as far as I am concerned! I look forward every year to growing my peppers, a great variety of which grow pretty well up here in the Pacific Northwest (last year I am grew six different varieties). According to this RealAge.com article, capsaicin may also inhibit the growth of cancer cells, ease pain, prevent heart attacks, kill bacteria that cause stomach ulcers, and more (website article[5])! Once again, Mother Nature comes through in a big way.

Another powerful spice to consider is ginger. I suffer from osteoarthritis, and during my book research I came across the idea to try ginger in my tea, which I have found helpful.

Ginger, when used regularly, is effective in relieving joint pain and arthritic symptoms.

(Ten Years Younger[46])

I am thinking here pineapple in my blender with a little shaved ginger root! This is something I have recommended to my eighty-three-year-old mother, as she also suffers from severe osteoarthritis in her hands, and I am implementing this in my diet as well right now to help with the daily fight I have with the never-ending pain in my thumbs.

With regard to arthritis, I recently read that olive oil can also be helpful due to its inherent anti-inflammatory properties. So not only is the Mediterranean Diet good for your heart, it may be helpful for your arthritis pain as well, so we don't have to take NSAIDs, which, as they did with me, can tear up the stomach and/or intestinal tract. I use olive oil now almost exclusively for cooking and I love the results; you can only use it on lower heat, eliminating the problem of cooking with the heat too high, which creates AGEs, one of our previously identified major aging enemies.

Spices and herbs are also rich in phytonutrients (discussed in the previous section) and they are, among many things, nature's most powerful beautifying agents. Examples are turmeric, curry (India has one of the lowest rates of Alzheimer's), cloves, allspice, sage, rosemary, oregano, thyme, ginger, mustard seed, parsley, basil, and marjoram (*Beautiful Brain, Beautiful You*[11]). Another aging authority lists what they believe are the best spices:

Anise, black pepper, caraway, cayenne, cinnamon, clove, coriander, cumin, fennel, fenugreek, licorice, marjoram, nutmeg, oregano, rosemary, saffron, sage, thyme and turmeric.

(SuperHealth[59])

So much to choose from, so little time! Like the lists of other anti-aging warriors/troops from the vegetables section, there are lots of spices out there for us to help ourselves in a completely natural way on our pathway to healthful and youthful longevity. Choose your weapons, bolster that savings account!

SECTION 3: LET'S EAT, DRINK, AND BE MERRY, OR NOT

BATTLE PLAN DIETS

Now let's talk about grouping the warriors and their weapons together in the form of diet plan troops that help us fight the fight against aging. I have never liked the word diet, because when I think of that word, I think of eating only grapefruit or drinking only liquids, etc., which is basically a severe calorie restriction way to *temporarily* lose weight. Now, as noted in *Prevention Positively Ageless,*[4] some calorie restriction (CR) does extend the lifespan of mice, yeast, worms, flies, and maybe the human species. The problem is, severe dieting overdoes this, and that stimulates the body to store more of the food you do eat in preparation for the next famine conditions, resulting in gaining even more weight every time whatever diet we are trying gets broken (*Healthy, Sexy, Happy*[28]). It becomes an ever-revolving door for many. I have always been so turned off at the word diet that I haven't ever actually done it, but I think many people have, as it gets a lot of media time.

So, staying away from the more common use of the diet concept, there are many books on this subject that take a different approach. It turns out that the word diet is defined as *habitual* nourishment; the kind and amount of food prescribed for a special reason. Thinking out loud, this definitely defines what we are discussing here as we look at the ways different aging experts talk about what to eat for longevity with youthfulness and health. I think I will call it the AGEDiet (aging gracefully effectively diet). Catchy. I think I like it, maybe it has some sticking power?

One healthy diet that takes a calorie restriction approach (used in a good way) came to me via a much-respected attorney friend of mine named Peter, who was excited about the book *Volumetrics Weight-Control: Feel Full on Fewer Calories*[35] and recommended that I take a look at it during my book research phase. The title may be a little misleading, though, because it is not about reducing volume of food; it is about maintaining the usual volume but eating foods with fewer calories for that volume, so you feel just as full but lose weight. Here are some of the high points of this idea:

- **Foods with lower energy density have fewer calories for the same weight.**

- **Fat is the most energy dense food element, alcohol second, then carbohydrates and protein, then water at zero.**

- Lean people have diets of lower energy density than obese individuals.

- People who stayed on a low-energy-dense weight loss plan maintained the lost weight in a two-year period.

- Water that's incorporated into food plays a crucial role in controlling hunger.

- An example of two foods with equal calories: twenty times as much tomato as pretzels.

Other aging authorities echo things that we have already discussed, such as these six:

☐ Eat real food—unprocessed, local/regional, seasonal and organic; don't eat fake food (e.g. sugar).
☐ Find your unique balance of protein, complex carbohydrates, and good fats at each meal.
☐ Eat breakfast.
☐ Don't skip meals or eat more than necessary.

❑ Have healthy snacks.
❑ Relax and enjoy your food; i.e., practice conscious eating.

(Winning at Aging[44])

While yet others talk in terms of diet and longevity:

Three Longevity Food Groups

1. *Antioxidant fruits and veggies.*
2. *Proteins, lean meats and healthy fats.*
3. *Whole grains, legumes, and other (unrefined) carbohydrates.*
(The Longevity Bible[42])

Or, foods to stay young naturally:

❑ Eat a minimum of five portions of fruits and veggies daily, up to nine if you can.
❑ Grow your own if you can.

- ☐ Pick your own fruit if you can.
- ☐ Eat local produce if you can.
- ☐ Keep chickens for eggs, if you can.
- ☐ Organic priorities: dairy, poultry and eggs, meat, apples and pears, raspberries and strawberries, cherries, nectarines and peaches, non-American grapes, celery and peppers, potatoes.
- ☐ Substitute a sweet potato for carbs—vitamins C and E boost the carotenoids' antioxidant capabilities.
- ☐ And: "One of the best, and cheapest, anti-aging tonics is to drink plenty of water." Body and brain need rehydration to function optimally.

(1001 Ways to Stay Young Naturally[39])

Or, just plain longevity foods:

1. Allium family of veggies (garlic, onion, chives, leeks, etc.)

2. Whey protein

3. Chili peppers

4. Cabbage-broccoli family

5. Carrots

6. Sweet potatoes, yams

7. Nuts and seeds

8. Medicinal mushrooms like shiitake, maitake, coriolus, reishi

9. "Green drinks"; i.e., powdered green drinks

10. Cold-water fish

11. Olive oil

12. Berries

13. Green peas

14. Bran cereals

15. Spices

16. Dark green, leafy veggies

17. Drink water

(The Metabolic Plan[78])

Anti-Aging Quick "Hot" Tip: Cold-water fish and extra-virgin olive oils and coconut oils help burn fat, but starchy foods do just the opposite, putting a "lock" on fat burning. (*Forever Young*[71])

Another battle plan diet example, from *Younger (Thinner) You Diet*,[33] tells us that we can reverse the effects of aging on muscles and bones by eating calcium-rich foods, fruits, veggies, beans, nuts and seeds, salmon, dairy products, and by drinking tea. WebMD reports a diet of *Fat-Fighting Foods*: Greek yogurt, quinoa, cinnamon, hot peppers, green tea, grapefruit, watermelon, pears and apples, grapes, berries, raw vegetables, sweet potatoes, eggs, coffee, oatmeal, crispbreads, tabbouleh, soup, salad, vinegar, nuts, air-popped popcorn, skim milk, lean meat, fish, and beans (website article[60]).

I am not trying to persuade you to habitually follow any one of these regimens solely. In fact, that does not make biologic sense to me, as each of us is unique and I think we are built for wide variety. I am recommending we each design our own customized AGEDiet that we not only will be able to continue, but will truly enjoy the journey all the while. This makes it likely that we will continue, which leads to more enjoyment, which makes continuance more likely. Now this is an ever-revolving door that is great to be stuck in! I want to give us all lots of things to choose from, with some basic understanding of how our choices impact our soma, and I am aligned with the philosophy (from both a biologic and a practical perspective) expressed here:

Discover the authentic diet that is uniquely right for you by removing suspicious food, then add them back and evaluate the effects of how you feel (i.e., experiment with the foods you eat).

(Winning at Aging[44])

I hope we each can create our own customized AGEDiet from all that the aging experts have to offer, and that we try new foods on for size every now and then because it keeps life, and eating, interesting.

EAT PALEO

Before we stop talking about our various diet battle plan choices, I want to talk separately about the Paleo diet. "Paleo" comes from the term Paleolithic and refers to our ancient ancestry, which intrigues me. I came across this, when I was compiling my aging authorities list of books to read, in the form of *The Paleo Solution*.[15] This book is one of the very few that I liked so much that I bought a copy for my library. The author does an excellent job of first describing how we digest foods, in great and easily understood scientific detail. He then proposes the Paleo solution, which is a diet that mimics the way our hunter-gatherer (HG) ancestors ate and the way they burned calories.

The Paleo-based diet really makes biologic sense to me. The book does a terrific job of explaining the very destructive role of gluten in our modern diets. The Paleo HG lifestyle concept has been a powerful influencer for me and a significant part of the food and exercise lifestyle changes I have undergone. Here's what the book says about eating Paleo:

- **Eat meat, wild fruits, fish, and shellfish; i.e., meals of protein, veggies, and fat, but no grains.**

- **Take or leave corn tortillas, rice.**

- Grains raise insulin levels, mess up your fatty acid ratios, irritate your gut, and are addictive, especially gluten-containing grains. Dairy and legumes have similar problems to grains.[15]

Here is another aging expert's opinion on some conditions for which we (hunter-gatherers) are designed:

- ☐ Eat nothing but whole, natural foods.
- ☐ Drink nothing but pure, clean water.
- ☐ Sleep all night.
- ☐ Keep active through most of the day.
- ☐ For optimal health, duplicate these simple behaviors as closely as possible.

(The Metabolic Plan[78])

Further perspective on this comes from *Healthy, Sexy, Happy*.[28] First, the current epidemic of gluten sensitivity is likely due to eating way too many refined grains in factory-food products. Second, one principle of a real, living food diet is to become a modern hunter-gatherer. According to Wikipedia, HG followers eat protein, fat, nonstarchy veggies, and carbohydrates, and they use herbs and spices. I practice what I preach here. I eat a lot Paleo; that is, I enjoy my meat supplemented with "colorful" veggies plus nuts and fruit as snacks; I eat more fish; I use a lot more olive oil and sometimes coconut oil; I eat very little bread and only minimal pasta or other grains; I eat only a little dairy and minimal processed foods; I use a lot of turmeric now, which I did not before; I work on using more spices in general, including one of my longtime favorites, cinnamon. I try to walk in my ancestors' shoes, as an extension of them, which I am (and you are).

One area in this discussion where consensus is lacking is whether we should eat whole grains (which many aging experts do recommend) or not eat grains at all, because most of them, including the whole grains, contain gluten (which our GI track isn't designed for, according to *The Paleo Solution*[15]). One of the exceptions to this is buckwheat, which is gluten-free and a great source of the calcium and fiber that are important to colon health and reducing blood sugar (*Ageless Face, Ageless Mind*[21]). Aging experts do seem to agree that "white" food—which refers to foods that are white and have been processed and refined, such as flour, rice pasta, bread, crackers, cereals, simple sugars like table sugar and high-fructose corn syrup, plus things made from those like soda pop and oh so many others—are *really* bad for us. But, the jury is still out on whole grains since there is no universal consensus. Myself, I like oatmeal and I occasionally eat whole grain toast, and I don't see enough consensuses to inspire me to give those up at this point.

In the end, I think we each should eat the types of foods that best suit our bodies. You can try different types of food programs to see what your body best responds to, customizing it to your individual needs and preferences. I believe that gluten is not good for us, but I am still drawn to whole grains. I would really recommend taking a more in-depth look at the HG lifestyle. It has a lot of validity, based on what I know and have learned.

Last, but not least, there are the "not to eat" foods. *Transcend: Nine Steps to Living Well Forever*[9] says to avoid trans fats in any amount, as they are unsafe, and recommends instead to get fat calories from omega-3. This aging authority says to eat salmon, trout, sardines, olive oil, avocados, and nuts. I hope by now that this is all starting to seem familiar and user-friendly to the reader. Other "infiltrator" foods and processes that need to be put on the avoid list are:

- **Whole milk products**

- **Fatty meats**

- **Avoid deep-frying**

- Keep oil at a moderate temperature to prevent free radicals

- Cut out sugar and refined starches

(Transcend: Nine Steps to Living Well Forever[9])

SECTION 4: THE DINING EXPERIENCE

Cooking is like love, it should be entered into with abandon, or not at all!

—Harriet Van Horne

I, like many, enjoy good food, but to make a food lifestyle change of the magnitude that I believe most of us need to make for our AGEDiet, we must find some pleasure in the process, enjoying the tangible and intangible reward side of cooking and eating. We have to be inspired to stay with it. We all know that change is not easy, and this may be the biggest, most important "battle" of them all! For instance, smell inspires me. I enjoy smelling as I cook, and I use my sense of smell to adjust my spice levels, instead of using taste. The aromas of cooking are very pleasurable to me, and the creativity of mixing various smells together entices me to cook.

I subscribe to cooking your own food being part of a healthy lifestyle, and here's something I heard recently that caught my attention: cook it yourself. Eat anything you want—as long as you are willing to cook it yourself. That is an interesting thought. Quite difficult to actually do, but it takes the eating healthy journey in the right direction, I think. In other words, if it has already been cooked and is now either frozen or canned or processed, that would not be part of an AGEDiet. Remember, 80 percent effort yields 95 percent results, so most anything is doable if we set our minds to it.

And it isn't only the cooking that can be rewarding, but the slow enjoyment of the food, dining with someone when you can, and savoring the whole experience, including the ambience around you; food can heal and renew; food can be your anti-aging medicine; enjoy the six tastes, eat consciously, and honor the signals of hunger and satiety (*Grow Younger, Live Longer*[53]).

Anti-Aging Quick Tip: Take twenty minutes to eat and lose weight without a complicated diet plan.

Eating slowly and savoring our food is good for us in more ways than one. WebMD (website link[5]) suggests setting a timer for twenty minutes to reinvent ourselves as a slow eater. They point out that this is one of the top habits for slimming down without a complicated diet plan (website article[22]). I try to do this but I have found it very hard. I can pretty easily get to fifteen minutes by putting my fork down often and chewing thoroughly, but twenty minutes has been difficult to achieve. Coming from a family of seven with often not enough food on the table, I blame my too-frequent speed-eating on making sure I got something to eat in the midst of all the chaos at dinnertime. But, like some of the other bits of expert advice, I think it takes us in the right direction on the aging gracefully pathway, and thank goodness, I recently heard that fifteen to twenty is ideal! I think it also improves digestion. Here is some additional expert input on the subject:

- ☐ Eat small amounts. Chew well.
- ☐ Eat slowly.
- ☐ Don't drink and eat in the same mouthful.
- ☐ Relax while you eat.

(The Metabolic Plan[78])

And, "Between mouthfuls, put down your knife and fork to savor flavors, [this] aids in digestion" (*1001 Ways to Stay Young Naturally*[39]). WebMD (website link[5]) echoes this, noting that most of us have a natural "eating pause" when we drop our fork for a couple of minutes, and if we watch for this, and don't take another bite, we are recognizing our quiet signal that we are full, but not stuffed (website article[22]). Sanjay Gupta, in his book *Chasing Life*,[95] tells us about the Okinawans who practice *hari hacha bu* (pushing back from the table before they are full, thus recognizing their quiet signal) and have lower rates of heart disease, stroke, and cancer. Plus, they have five times the number of centenarians as the United States. Their diet is also rich in fruits and vegetables and unrefined carbohydrates, and they eat fish several times per week.

Others give us some basic overriding concepts to frame our eating:

1. Eat primarily during the day.

2. Try to have the largest meal between one and three in the afternoon.

3. Make sure to drink enough fluids.

4. Eat a light dinner of veggies because they are easily digested.

5. Eat no later than seven p.m. because you will sleep better.

(Gary Null's Power Aging[77])

Anti-Aging Quick Tip: Dine well, stay fit, keep laughing, and enjoy life and the people you share it with. (*Age Proof Your Body*[47])

CHAPTER 4:

BURNING THE FUEL THAT FEEDS THE FLAME

SECTION 1: BURN, BABY, BURN

Exercise is the secret to great health. It is the great key to aging.

(Younger Next Year[36])

By now, the brain may be tuning out and nearly on information overload. Fear not, as the hard part is done! The most difficult and complex information has come before, and what we have left to look at is simpler in nature and in detail. That is not to say less important, however, because aging gracefully is a complex interaction of many things, not the least among them being exercise, rest, and the spirit. But, 80 percent of the penned portion of this book is now completed. The remaining 20 percent will be easier for us, with the last few pages being the tips and tidbits on aging that I uncovered in my literature research but that were not woven into the book's verbiage.

I share these in this way because, in the end, I didn't want to leave out any of the authoritative advice I sifted out from the aging literature, and it provides a place in the book where the bits of aging expert advice "pop" off the page in all their unadorned glory. For some, that may be the highlight of reading this book. Some may only read that section. I leave it up to the reader to decide how to make the book work for him/her in the best possible way.

This chapter is about burning calories. This is such a commonly discussed and well-understood subject that I will paint a fairly general picture from the aging authorities, with a dash of their creative thinking on exercising thrown in. The same holds true for the next chapter on the role of rest and relaxation. In part 3, we will look at the loftier subject of the spiritual/soul aspect of aging, again with very broad strokes and simplicity.

One of eight keys to longevity: Keep up regular physical activity.

(The Longevity Prescription[1])

We learned in part 2, chapter 2 that physical inactivity is one of the major aging accelerators. Let's look now at some options for fighting that aging enemy. There are two types of troops to burn the fuel that we intake in the form of food and drink. One is a fired-up metabolism so that we burn more calories. The other is any form of physical activity, exercise, or physical exertion (PEP, from now on) that burns calories. I think most of us, if not all, need both approaches to help us deal with excess weight as we age, and we need a big bag of calorie-burning choices to keep it interesting and effective so that we stay with it. I know for certain that I do, especially with my propensity for absorbing more fat and having a slower metabolism in my genetic makeup (more on that subject in a bit).

I do use both of these troops and their weaponry, and I use them whenever and as often as I can because every calorie I burn is that much less fat around my waist, upper arms, back, thighs, etc. There are a couple of terms that are important to define before we begin this conversation: periodization and cross-training. Periodization is the process of varying a training program at regular time intervals to bring about optimal gains in physical performance. Cross-training is typically defined as an exercise regimen that uses several modes of training. We will discuss both of these in detail as we "move" along.

TROOPS FIRED UP AND READY TO GO

Starting with firing up our metabolism, *O Magazine* dedicated its May 2012 issue to "How to Get Better with Age." One of the articles included in that issue was "Turn Up the Burn"[88] by RealAge cofounder Dr. Mehemet Oz, who starts by saying that ***extra years bring extra pounds but it doesn't have to be that way.*** To help with that, he shares tips on ways to turn up the burn. Here is his list of certain activities, foods, and beverages (he also included a few supplements that I have an innate bias against, so in full disclosure, I left those off) that can fire up our metabolism, burning more calories:

- **First thing yoga: can double your metabolic rate first thing in the morning.**

- **Drink cold water, as it may spike metabolism by 30 percent for as long as an hour. Also may force your body to use energy to warm it.**

- **Eat a protein-packed breakfast: takes more energy to digest than carbs or fat.**

- Enjoy a cup of coffee: keeps metabolic rate humming.

- Go for a walk.

- Snack on tahini dip (made from sesame seeds, which improve metabolism and curb appetite).

- Chew a stick of sugarless gum.

- Go for a brisk fifteen-minute walk.

- Spice up lunch with peppers (capsaicin, the key substance that makes chili peppers hot, stimulates your "fight or flight" stress response and may increase metabolism by 23 percent. Peppers may even improve your muscle-to-fat ratio: research suggests that capsaicin inhibits the generation of fat cells).

- Cook dinner with coconut oil: it is rapidly converted into energy and may bump metabolism by 12 percent.

- Do two to three thirty-minute strength-training sessions each week, as muscle burns more energy.

- Use your muscles with your mind (visualizing a workout can trick your mind into strengthening your calorie-zapping muscle).

- Sip a cup of green tea: a greater boost in metabolism than caffeine alone.

- Add dairy: calcium binds to fat to reduce absorption, and in the bloodstream, excess calcium helps break down fat cells.

- Garnish with dill weed or chives: flavonoids increase production of thyroid hormones, which boost metabolism.

- Unwind with a glass of wine: alcohol can raise the metabolic rate for up to ninety-five minutes.

- Get regular sleep to prevent disruption of circadian rhythms.

Dr. Oz finishes his article with his thoughts on four things to turn back the clock:

- Limit sweets.

- Go outside (get sun for vitamin D: need ten to fifteen minutes, three times per week).

- Take five (lower stress, as those with higher stress appear at least a decade older than low-stress-level counterparts).

- Get romantic.

Anti-Aging Quick Tip: Green tea can really rev up calorie burning.

Dr. Oz's list is very thorough and complete, based on my book research findings. THANK YOU, Dr. Oz! Other aging authorities echo these items, such as WebMD with regard to the value of green tea, pointing out that some studies have suggested that drinking green tea can not only rev up the body's calorie-burning engine temporarily, but it includes a bonus: it does this without any extra calories (website article[22]). It's a twofer! We also learned in the previous chapter that teamed up, green tea and the spice turmeric enhance each other's health-giving properties and may help reverse cellular aging. This simple, inexpensive green tea/turmeric aging tidbit with great return on investment is an ideal example of the kind of information I found to be so valuable when researching and writing this book. Let's have a cup of green tea (I prefer a green and white tea blend because it is a little smoother) to get fired up and ready to go!

SECTION 2: HOOKED ON A FEELING

Now, the second way to burn more fuel is definitely harder, requiring a lot of self-discipline and commitment and, well, physical effort. It is *so* tough sometimes to work up the energy to get up and get going, to use some of the calorie-burning and muscle-burning troops that are available. I can relate, as can anyone who includes exercise in his/her lifestyle. When I got home from work after a long, hard day, I used to have to fight with myself over getting some exercise in. Even since retirement, I still sometimes do battle with myself to take the time and get some physical activity accomplished. I don't always have the "pep" to do any PEP!

But do you know what I have found? I have found that if I self-talk myself into the idea, somewhere in the process I start feeling better physically and more positive mentally, which helps reinforce the next point of choice, to do or not to do. When I was running, we called it "runner's high." It would be very difficult to run at first, but all of a sudden, the euphoria would kick in and it became a very pleasurable experience to keep running.

(At least up to twenty miles, where most of us "hit the wall" and have to keep running by sheer willpower pitted against physical pain, which I learned in my one and only marathon—but I digress.)

I think these same positive feelings, which are linked to the release of endorphins in our brain, can come from many, if not all, forms of exercise if we stick with them long enough and are paying attention to what our body is trying to tell us. It is our soma's system for reinforcing a behavior that is in actuality good for us. This is good. This is good. Keep it up…I think you see what I mean. *1001 Ways to Stay Young Naturally*[39] notes: regular exercise is key—it plays an essential role in anti-aging and stress reduction, better moods, more energy, less insomnia. *Between a Rock and a Hot Place*[82] notes that "it [exercise] also helps with depression."

I have definitely personally experienced many of the attributes of exercise, which are very motivational for me. I am a type A personality who needs to deal with the stresses I create for myself, who also needs lots of energy for my always long and never-ending to-do list, who needs to sleep well at night, and yes, who strives to age as gracefully as possible—sound familiar? Does the shoe fit? Well, if not, try it again, taking it slowly at first. We are physically and biologically designed for PEP, and we do not fare well without it.

Anti-Aging Quick Tip: "Exercise does all the right things for the biochemistry, the body, and the mind." (*Longevity Made Simple*[51])

A good friend convinced me to start exercising regularly when I was just thirty. We were runners then (before the knees and hips said "no more concrete, no more asphalt, no more"). I balked at first, but once I tried it, I became hooked. That feeling of euphoria I got after a few minutes kept me going back for more, including my one and only marathon, for which I proudly and visibly display my medal for making it to the finish line. I take note of it occasionally to remind me of the achievement and to remind myself not to do it again—once was truly enough for me; I merely wanted to prove I could pass that ultimate runner's test. I am one of those people who actually enjoyed running and I still miss it today, so sometimes I jog over to the gym to satisfy that desire to run. The yearning still drives me to try, so I do, but in short spurts now, because I really don't want to have to go see my high school classmate orthopedic surgeon about that knee.

In addition, there is also the feeling of pride and joy in achievement when I am done exercising and the reinforcement when I can see visible improvement, in any shape or form, especially if it is part of my body's shape! It always feels *so* good, both physically and mentally, when I am done. I saw an uncredited post on Facebook one time about staying in it, day by day, inch by inch, each rep, every workout, each failure, and doing it when we don't feel like it, which gets us closer to our goal. Yes, it does.

> One of the best ways to reverse the all-too-common effects of aging is to move well and use your whole body: You can have a spring in your step, an air of grace and stability and ease of movement at any age. The more you move, the better off you are.
>
> (Change Your Age[43])

When I couldn't run anymore, it got tougher to keep a regular exercise program going. For a few years I did dance aerobics at home, then I tried Pilates, which I found very hard to do with only a videotape and me, myself, and I. Pilates was definitely an "instructor" type of exercise for me, but I didn't belong to a gym back then, so, not being able to do it the way it was supposed to be done, I lost interest. Unfortunately, over time I slipped into the easy pattern of exercising less frequently, finally reaching the point of not doing any formal exercise program at all not too long after that big fiftieth birthday. I was soon to discover this was very bad timing, as menopause was commencing, and with it would come increased belly fat and decreased metabolism. One fateful morning, the lack of exercise caught up with me. In 2005, at age fifty-four, when I stepped on the scale I gasped, because somehow I had gradually added on weight until I was now carrying 168 pounds—on my small-boned frame and being only five feet four and a half inches tall. Apparently, I had also stopped stepping on the scale...

Yikes! Imagine that, carrying thirty extra pounds around every day, all day long, twenty-four/seven! Well, I didn't have to imagine it because I created and was living with it. I knew I had to do something, but I still resisted a regular exercise program, choosing instead to try to lose the weight by adjusting calories, such as reducing my beverage and "calorie rich" food intake and increasing my weeding in the garden (which can be problematic in the Northwest, since it is not much fun weeding in the rain that falls about two-thirds of the year around here).

But by the summer of 2006, I had made some real progress, having lost almost twenty-five pounds, and I was wearing clothes that I had not been able to wear in a while. This was very reinforcing for me. I soon learned, however, that I could not keep the weight off with that program, and it started creeping back up. By early 2007 it became abundantly clear that regular exercise, as it had been in the past, needed to be part of my aging gracefully future. When I couldn't seem to get an exercise rhythm going, but kept lamenting about the need to do it, my husband, Morris, suggested I look at the YMCA gym near our home. I pursued it and found it very appealing, with a great variety of exercise options and classes to keep me enthusiastic and committed about going there, all for a very reasonable price tag.

I was in part motivated that particular year by the fact that I had been accepted to go back to school at the University of Washington for my MBA degree, starting fall quarter. It was even more motivational once I met my classmates, as my entire class was younger than I, many by twenty years or more! I wanted to fit in, to wear "hip" clothes (which I got my sister, Janice, who has always been very hip, to help me shop for), and to be in sync with these young classmates of mine.

For the start of this "rebirthing" of my exercise routine, I focused initially on doing aerobics four to six days a week. I also bought myself an iPod Nano and filled it with my music favorites to listen to while I worked out. Music and exercise truly go well together for me, moving the whole thing up the enjoyment scale by several notches. A year or so after I joined the gym, I got my weight back down to 139 pounds, close to my marriage weight of 135.

Again, unfortunately, after a while I seemed to be getting less and less out of my gym time, which didn't make much sense to me at first. Then I heard and read about the importance of doing more than only aerobics, so I cut one day of aerobics and substituted strength training (weights). Two years ago last September, I added a yoga class two times per week to improve my balance and flexibility, reducing my aerobic exercise to two or three days per week.

Sometimes on nice days, instead of going to the gym, I push the wheelbarrow around or weed my garden for exercise and a little vitamin D, and to shake things up in the physical exertion troops. I benefit, and so do my yard and my gardens. I have found that I enjoy this mix of PEP a lot more than doing aerobic exercise alone. This is my version of cross-training. The mix also allows me to get creative and change up what kind of exercise and physical exertion weaponry I choose to do on any given day. In my yoga class, our instructor never does the same routine twice. I am confident that she knows about and believes in the concept of cross-training. Making use of that idea for my workouts keeps my body from figuring out my routine and becoming more efficient as a result, because that would mean I would have to ratchet up how hard I work to burn the same amount of calories. It also keeps it more interesting and allows my creative juices to flow and enhance my results.

Once I get my exercise routine going, I try to make the best use of my time by concentrating on using multiple muscle groups during exercise, good posture, and a good pace alternated with a slower pace (periodization), so I can get the most "burn" out of the time and energy spent. When my posture is good, I feel like I get a lot more out of whatever exercise activity I am doing, not to mention how much posture affects our age appearance, as we talked about way back in the beginning of this book. There are some good reasons for considering posture and muscle groups when exercising as noted on the website RealAge.com (website link[3]):

- **Keep your gaze at eye level.** This simple move prevents neck strain.

- **Relax those hunched shoulders.** Drop your shoulders as low as they comfortably go.

- **Lift your chest** *slightly*—not into a military stance with chest thrust out and shoulders way back. This helps prevent rounded shoulders.

- **Lengthen your spine.** Imagine a string pulling the top of your head up to the ceiling to improve your posture.

- **Tighten your abs.** Strong abs help support your lower back.

- **Don't lock your knees.** Keep knees slightly bent. Also, keep your toes lined up to prevent overstressing your knees.

- **Breathe.** Count reps out loud to avoid holding your breath. As you inhale, relax your lower abs and fill your chest. As you exhale, suck in your abs to force air out.

- **Keep moving between exercises.** It keeps your heart rate up.

- **As you get stronger, work out more.**

- **With cardio, go a little longer.**

- **With weights, add more reps or use slightly heavier weights in your weight training routine.** Again, slightly. Use proper form to stay injury-free.

Let me share more detail about my personal periodization. On the elliptical or treadmill I change the inclination, and/or I change the resistance up and down often (and with variable amounts of time at each level) during any given day's routine to vary which muscles I am exercising during my changeable time program of twenty-five to thirty-five minutes. I also pedal forward or backward or both for variation. I vary which machine I use, the time of day I exercise, and whether I have eaten anything before I start. When I do my one day of weight training, I vary the number of reps and/or the amount of weight I am trying to push around.

Many of the aging experts support this variable approach as to what kind, and what intensity, of workout we do as being very important, verifying that it prevents the body from developing the efficiencies we recently talked about, which increases how many calories we burn. It also helps prevent burnout of our exercise routine, and may even help prevent injury by using different muscle groups on different days and at differing intensities, spreading the load around and keeping our bodies balanced.

I recently evolved to using a "HIIT" program as least once or twice a week in substitution for one or two aerobics workouts, but still in addition to my two yoga classes and a weight-lifting session. HIIT stands for high-intensity interval training. It means alternating bursts of intense activity with intervals of lighter activity. This is another example of periodization. For me, this is mostly on the elliptical, which is gentle on my hips and knees that I am carefully protecting to try to avoid joint replacement surgery, as I talked about in the prologue. Occasionally I will use the treadmill for variation.

The genetic testing that I first mentioned in part 2, chapter 2 and again earlier in this chapter, was a big influencer here. Really bad genetic test news: my report for weight management said that with my genetic pattern I am less able to break down body fat in response to exercise, so I will tend to lose *less* weight and body fat than expected with moderate exercise.

More bad genetic news: I tend to absorb more dietary fat and have a slower metabolism. Bad, bad combination! Now that does not seem fair! I absorb fat easily and don't respond as well to exercise. Yikes. No wonder it has been such a struggle for these last few years to see weight loss, in spite of all the PEP I do. I am guessing many others have this same kind of genetic "bad" weight gain combination of lower metabolism and being somewhat unresponsive to exercise. It explains a lot for me with regard to myself and our overweight American society. The final conclusion "positive spin" on the report was that I am in the category of responsive to fat restriction and more responsive to high-intensity exercise. So, I must keep those French fries to a bare minimum and regularly HIIT myself, as my best shot at weight control lies therein.

> **Anti-Aging Quick Tip: Work out before breakfast: "Training on an empty stomach turns on some interesting genetic machinery that is important not only in fat loss but also longevity." (*The Paleo Solution*[15])**

Getting in one or two workouts each week before breakfast has become a big priority since I started writing this book. As *The Paleo Solution*[15] noted, there is the duo benefit to this of fat loss and longevity, not to mention it really gets my day off on the right foot. With all this I have been fairly successful at keeping my weight down around 141–145 pounds, give or take a holiday or discipline lapse "five pound or so gain" along the way that I beat back eventually.

I am determined not to let the upward trajectory weight gain with age become inevitable, which I think about pretty much every day now (of course, writing this book is playing a role here, too). This is a point in our aging gracefully journey where that mirror reevaluation comes in handy. It isn't always pretty, but it *is* always motivational for me once I work up the willingness/courage to look. No one said it was going to be easy. It isn't. But, it is packed with value for us. Great investment return!

SECTION 3: MOTIVATION/ INSPIRATION

Think of your workouts as important meetings you have scheduled with yourself. Bosses don't cancel.

(Uncredited)

Speaking of motivational, motivators can be either internal or external. As I said earlier, when I exercise more regularly, and more effectively, I note that I have more energy and can fit into clothes I haven't been able to wear in a while. This is both externally (wearing old clothes) and internally (having more energy) motivational. That external motivator provides a whole new wardrobe without spending any money! Seeing often a favorite article of clothing that we love but can't wear can be a powerful driver.

As I mentioned earlier in the book, WebMD (website link[5]) suggested hanging that favorite dress or a smokin' pair of jeans where we can see them every day, so we can keep our eyes on the prize (website article[22]). Once we can wear that prize, we can pick another as a new goal for further progress, and so on! Right now for me it is a favorite linen blouse that is a little too snug once buttoned, so I have it hanging where I see it every time I go into our closet, to remind me of how important my fat restriction and HIIT exercise are. (I do take Sundays off, though, as a day of rest.)

Another motivating idea I came up with recently is to print a picture from the web or cut out one from a magazine of an outfit "to die for" that requires some change in weight and body shape to wear it the way it was meant to be worn. I posted it in plain sight in front of my desk so that I see it often. I found a great one on the web—a salmon pink two-piece summer dress with pinkish gray sling-back heels and a matching purse. I love looking at it and daydreaming of wearing it sometime soon.

It is clear to me that I need motivators, because I find it hard to keep up the five to six exercise events a week, week after week, month after month. It is much easier not to do it. This need I have is proven theory, since I sometimes lapse and gain that five or so back. My track record in this department isn't as consistent as I would like, unfortunately. The good news is, I am also pretty consistent about getting back on track after my lapses.

I am thinking that I am not alone with this issue and that most (maybe all) of us need these internal and external motivators to balance out the negatives. I have mentioned some of the ones that I use, but I think we need a *big* basket of motivators to choose from. The key is to find the one(s) that work best for the individual, customizing this part of our lifestyle, as we did for what we eat. Let's consider a few additional possible motivators.

Anti-Aging Quick Tip: An extra pound of muscle added burns seventy-five calories a day to maintain. If we add a pound of fat instead of muscle, we only need two calories a day to maintain that extra body mass. (*Low-Fat Living*[8])

So, ANY amount of muscle we gain burns almost forty times as many calories as any fat we gain! That's a darn good return on investment. Speaking of muscle mass to burn calories, it is important to realize, as noted by one of the aging experts (*Ten Years Younger*[46]), that there are also things that can erode muscle mass: insulin resistance, increased cortisol, too much inflammation, a decline in hormones—sound familiar? Do you hear voices from chapter 2 calling? These aging enemies are bad actors in more ways than one! Not only do they age us directly, but they make it hard to keep our weight down, and we know that excess weight ages us and may lead to insulin resistance, inflammation, etc., which leads to less muscle and likely weight gain, which leads to... It is a "circular" battle that feeds on itself. Breaking that circular battle is key to aging gracefully.

Muscle mass is your anti-aging ally. Fitness keeps you young.[46]

The routine mix of PEP and motivators that I am using now seems to be a good mix and balance for me. I am far enough along that I have started to take pride in some fairly nicely sculpted shoulders and upper arms that I don't mind showing off when that the weather is warm enough. I have set my ultimate weight goal at my 135-pound marriage weight, but I am not there yet, and I know trying on my wedding dress at this point would not be the pretty sight that it was almost twenty years ago. Once that linen blouse and dream outfit in the picture works for me, I am going to unpack that dress as the ultimate "prize." I still have weight fluctuations depending on what I eat and how much I exercise. *No excuse, I know better, obviously!* But, I have that ultimate goal in clear sight, and because I can envision it, I believe I will in fact get there.

MORE MOTIVATORS

Here is another possible motivator: "Overall mortality falls with exercise" (*Younger Next Year: A Guide to Living Like 50 Until*

You're 80 and Beyond[36]). Or if that one is not powerful enough, here's another from Swedish researchers in 2005: "Those who had engaged in robust physical activity at least two times per week since their youth or middle age had a 50% lower chance of developing dementia and a 60% lower risk of developing Alzheimer's than those who were sedentary" (*Juicy Living, Juicy Aging*[50]).

Fitbie.com had an article (website article[25]) sharing that a review of studies on cognitive function showed that those with a normal weight performed better on executive functions like meeting goals, making decisions, and planning ahead. I like this one a lot. It speaks so loud and clear to me. I was born to organize, and I love planning and making projects come to fruition from ground zero, so these executive functions are extremely important and valuable to me. I know that I need to keep those around for the long haul because I would not be me without them.

Anti-Aging Quick Tip: From a *USA Today* article: For the cost of a walk a day, you might be able to put off or avoid altogether taking blood pressure drugs or cholesterol medications, for which you could spend fifty dollars to one hundred dollars or more a month. (Juicy Living, Juicy Aging[50])

Avoid developing diabetes and you could see much bigger savings. The cost per person averages more than thirteen thousand dollars a year. And if you can stave off dementia and live on your own longer, you can avoid the seventy thousand dollars or more a year that nursing homes cost.[50] And, guess what? People who exercise regularly keep burning calories at a higher rate for several hours after (*Volumetrics Weight-Control*[35]), so regularity is very important here, as it is in many things, such as—might I say again—brushing and flossing! When I am on track, the regularity is self-perpetuating for me because it is the quickest way to see visible progress in the mirror and on the scale.

Or, how about this from *Rethinking Aging*[13] For every ten pounds you lose, you ask 30–50 percent less of your knees with each heel strike and spare your bunions. I relate to this one only too well, as my right foot bunion can barely handle a low-heeled shoe now, and cannot take some of my shoes for more than a few minutes at my current weight of 144. Yet, I daydream of wearing true heels again, as I love how they look with everything from jeans to a favorite formal gown or wedding dress!

Rethinking Aging[13] also tells us, which makes complete bio-logic sense, that we are better off postponing decrepitude or diminishing its intensity than we are trying to recover function once it has set in—not to mention the heavy price we pay both monetarily and otherwise if we wait until it does. As I always told my patients, prevention is less expensive, more predictable, and far less painful than treatment to fix the problem once it develops!

Speaking of paying a price, that concept reminds me to share again one of my favorite quotes (my wording) from my mentor, Dr. Saul Schluger: no matter our choices, there will always be a price to be paid. The question we have to ask, and answer, is will the outcome be worthy of the price. If it is, do it. If the outcome is not worthy of the price, then choose another path. Dr. Schluger was talking about periodontal therapy choices for patients, but I have always felt that this applied to all aspects of my life, and have used it many, many times over these thirty-plus years during my self-talk when faced with a difficult decision. It certainly applies to a regular PEP routine, which is clearly way more valuable than the price paid. Enough said on that subject.

Or a last, but far from least, possible motivator, *exercise is a key to maintaining our independence as we get older.* This one also strikes a very harmonic chord with me. I plan to still be in my beautiful home on our secluded hilly acre of Northwest wooded property when I move on from this life. Sadly, in the last few years, I have seen several, very personal, very gut-wrenching, and very real examples of what happens when mobility is lost, and the extent to which that ratchets up a dependence on others, and on equipment like walkers and wheelchairs.

It can sometimes even be fatal, as in the case of the pulmonary embolism (secondary to being wheelchair-bound due to a leg fracture from osteoporosis) that took my baby sister's life at only age fifty-four two years ago. This loss still tugs at my heart strings, and the experience "video" of watching her declining independence over those last few years before her death is permanently etched in my mind. Its presence serves as another motivator for me.

1001 Ways to Stay Young Naturally[39] adds that we even want to keep our wrists and ankles mobile to make independent life more likely into old age. Clearly, we do need these wrists and ankles, and like my thumbs with their minimal grip strength, we will miss them the most when we don't have them anymore. It is so easy to take our various body parts for granted, but I now see clearly how important it is to keep in the forefront of our mind the important contribution that all our various body parts make in our lives and on our aging gracefully pathway. We are the keeper and the maintainer of the vessel and all its appendages. We must honor the responsibility to take great care of it. I believe this is part of our life's lesson. As Betty Ford said: "Don't compromise yourself. You are all you've got." I couldn't agree more.

Exercise for the young is an option, but exercise for the old is a must.

(Living Longer for Dummies[57]*)*

SECTION 4: MOVE 'EM OUT

Now that we are motivated, the next logical question is, what kind of exercise is best? I started this conversation somewhat already with my personal exercising story. I and the aging authorities agree pretty much across the board with *The Longevity Bible*[42] that aerobics (cardiovascular conditioning) alone is not enough; balance/flexibility training (like yoga or similar), and strength (weight) training are also necessary. I like to think of this as the exercise triangle for aging well. Relative to the aerobics part, some believe, like *The Metabolic Plan*[78] and *The Paleo Solution*,[15] that we, truth be told, need high-intensity interval training like that of our ancestors' lifestyle. My genetic testing certainly says that I do!

We are hunter-gatherers (HG's): Fitness was a foraging life-style but with much downtime and relaxation. HG's lived active, vigorous life: We are literally "born to be fit." Best? Cross-training and periodization (those planned changes in exercise to avoid burnout and foster progress.) Recommend strength training,

*interval training to be strong, flexible,
have muscle mass and optimize hormones.*

(The Paleo Solution[15])

Resharing the conditions for which we (hunter-gatherers) are designed:

- ❏ Eat nothing but whole, natural foods.
- ❏ Drink nothing but pure, clean water.
- ❏ Sleep all night.
- ❏ Keep active through most of the day.

*For optimal health, duplicate these simple
behaviors as closely as possible.*

(The Metabolic Plan[78])

We also can use to our advantage a need to do routine chores, because these can be significant calorie-burning activities that give us the exertion benefit with the bonus that it gets some of

our chores done. I respond well to this kind of immediate reinforcement. RealAge.com offers the following table in their article
"Double-Duty Exercise Opportunities" (website article[24]):

Top ten household chores for burning calories*

1. Moving furniture	225 calories
2. Scrubbing floors	189 calories
3. Raking leaves	171 calories
4. Gardening	162 calories
5. Mowing the lawn	162 calories
6. Washing the car	153 calories
7. Cleaning windows	153 calories
8. Vacuuming	84 calories
9. Washing dishes	76 calories
10. Doing laundry	72 calories

*Estimations based on a 150-pound
person and thirty minutes of activity.

Now that is something I can, and do, make use of often, as
I am a neat-and-order kind of person, not to mention that it is
another "change things up" opportunity, with a clean house or
car to boot! And, if I turn on some up-tempo music and speed up
the activity, I know I can burn even more calories. It is a twofer

way that all of us can get workouts into our busy schedule. This is my kind of creative thinking! Some aging experts, like *Juicy Living, Juicy Aging*,[50] provide other interesting alternatives to traditional exercise troops and weaponry:

New "juicy" exercises:

- ❐ Boxing
- ❐ Tai Chi
- ❐ Creative Movement
- ❐ Trampoline
- ❐ Tango
- ❐ Counting Steps
- ❐ Gyrokenesis (a group exercise with flow and rhythm essential)
- ❐ Kettlebell Training (combines dumbbell training with high-intensity cardio)
- ❐ Capoeria (Brazilian martial art)
- ❐ BalleCore (integrates Pilates, hatha yoga, and ballet)

What is the bottom line? It is clear that we need exercise more as aged than we did when we were young, and that the benefits are well worth those tough days. As said so well in an uncredited quote I saw recently on Facebook: "It's not going to be easy. It's going to be worth it." That is a fantastic mantra for our aging gracefully pathway. Regular PEP is definitely **not** easy, but it is indeed **worth it**! And, as pointed out in *RealAge*,[26] the whole point is to promote a healthy, vibrant and young old age—e.g., being eighty with the energy and vigor of a fifty-five-year-old. I believe this is achievable with the right mix in the aging "cocktail." My question is, can we make it fun, too, at least some of the time?

We don't stop playing because we grow old. We grow old because we stop playing.

—George Bernard Shaw

I love that quote. "Play" can be a good exercise alternative to help us mix things up so we keep our bodies guessing what's next. It doesn't have to be a gym routine every day, or a freshly mowed lawn or sparkling scrubbed floor. *Looking After Your Body: An Owner's Guide to Successful Aging*[56] offers some other fun choices:

Your Workout Made Easy

- ☐ Play ball with your grandkids.
- ☐ Walk to the store to get a newspaper versus delivery.
- ☐ Take the dog out for an extra walk each day or cover hillier terrain.
- ☐ Dust off your bicycle.
- ☐ Take two extra turns around the mall when you shop.
- ☐ Chose the farthest parking spot and let your legs do the rest.
- ☐ Walk the golf course.
- ☐ Rake leaves.
- ☐ Stretch and strengthen your ankles when you watch TV.

We also don't have to even *go* to a gym to get beneficial physical exertion. WebMD (website link[5]) shows you how to exercise simply at home because, as they say, your own body weight and gravity can do the job without machines or dumbbells. If you have ever tried a triceps pushup or forearm plank (which I learned in yoga), you understand the concept of using body weight and gravity to help make exercising accessible in your living room or anywhere. We can even exercise while waiting in line: suck in the abs for ten seconds and release until your wait is over and you have done ab toning, burning a few extra calories while you waited!

Think of it this way: it doesn't require a special place to get good physical exertion, it requires our having the impetus to do that first step, pose, weight pull, etc., and being creative about our calorie-burning choices. At the end of this conversation on burning calories, it is all about winning the aging war. With all the PEP troops and weaponry that we have as options, we can win this physical activity battle. Keep it up. This is good. Keep it up.

As a final thought in this chapter on exercise, here are another eight reasons from *Winning at Aging*[44] why physical activity needs to be a daily part of our lifestyle:

☐ Exercise ignites the spark in life.
☐ It increases longevity.
☐ It strengthens heart and lungs.
☐ It stimulates the brain.

- ❑ It reduces stress.
- ❑ It strengthens the immune system.
- ❑ It balances blood sugar.
- ❑ It strengthens muscles and bones.

There is no shortage of great reasons and ways to exercise, to be physically active, or to physically exert ourselves as we were designed to do. All good stuff. All good for us. Enough PEP talk.

CHAPTER 5:

HEALING TIME

SECTION 1: THE BODY AT REST, RELAXED

SLEEPYTIME

According to *Grow Younger, Live Longer*,[53] there are two kinds of deep rest: restful sleep and restful awareness. This is a way of thinking that I had not considered before I worked on this book. I thought in terms of actual sleep as our only rest, but not true. We will take a look at both of these, starting with sleep.

Anti-Aging Quick Tip: Sleeping enough adds two or more years to your life. (website article[16])

One of the proven keys to a long healthy life is sleep. Healthy at 100,[14] along with many other aging authorities, echoes this idea, stating that getting enough sleep is a longevity step. Jane Fonda, who is a phenomenal example of aging gracefully, agrees in her book on aging, *Prime Time.*[85] But sleep can be elusive for many of us. I know that I struggle at times to stay asleep, often waking during the night with night sweats since menopause began more than ten years ago. My nature is not to take medications if I can help it, so I have never used hormone replacement therapy (HRT) or any of the sleep prescriptions. I certainly have been tempted to talk to my internist about it a few times, but ultimately I always come back to the idea that I want to let my body deal naturally with sleep and rest issues by trying to hear and understand what it needs, then trying to provide that.

*The more you understand—and listen
to—your personal clock (circadian rhythm),
the more rested you feel.*

(Healthy Aging for Dummies[81])

Now that I am only on a fixed-time workday when I fulfill my position as an affiliate associate professor, I am able to let my body tell me when to go to bed and when to wake up at least most days, which has resulted in feeling more rested, but it is still sometimes a struggle to get fully restful sleep. This is one of my aging battles that I don't win every night, but not for lack of trying.

I have noticed, however, there are things that work for me in contributing to a good night's sleep, such as days when I have pushed the wheelbarrow up and down our hilly property a few times, or have weeded in my garden or yard for hours on end. From *The 100 Year Lifestyle*[31] comes a similar message. To sleep well, try:

*Power walking. Pilates. Gardening. Yoga.
Sauna. [I would add steam or warm bath/
Jacuzzi.] Drink lots of water.*

Certain foods may also help us get the sleep we need. As noted in 5 *Foods That Help You Sleep Better* on the RealAge website (website link[3]), consider almonds, bananas, skim milk, oatmeal, or whole-wheat bread, or mix and match for a good night's sleep. The article concludes by noting that six to nine hours of sleep per night can reduce your RealAge by 0.9 to 1.5 years. I am all over that!

Interestingly, one tidbit that I found in *Forever Young*[71] tells us that the opposite of sleep, sleep deprivation, causes us to overeat. According to WebMD (website link[5]) and a University of Michigan researcher, sleeping an extra hour could help us drop fourteen pounds of weight a year, because it replaces idle activities such as snacking (website article[22]). So, sleeping too little can add weight, whereas sleeping a little longer helps drop weight. Our work is cut out for us, but the aging gracefully path is clear. We need good sleep time, like we need good PEP time.

Sleep (and exercise) also stimulates growth hormone, allowing more collagen and elastin production, which is good for our skin's appearance (*You Being Beautiful*[93]). Hence the term "beauty sleep"! I always thought this was just another one of my mother's funny sayings. Not true, it is reality in the form of better skin. Bet you didn't think of that phrase in a reality sense; I know that I didn't. Oh, that mother's voice again in my brain, and right after all. Darn. And it took me all this research to come to that conclusion. Darn. All told, there are plenty of good reasons to work at getting enough sleep hours in each night.

RELAXED

Very closely related to sleep is relaxation, also called restful awareness or mindfulness. This can come in many forms, and of course, as with all these aging bits of advice, the key is finding what suits the individual best. One of the easy relaxation methods is mindful meditation, where you get comfortable, close your eyes, and focus on your breathing for seven minutes or so. Drs. Oz and Roizen talk about this in a RealAge "tip" (website link[3]). Those seven minutes are not only good for the mind, but it can help control cravings, help us eat less, and get thin (woo-hoo). It is also very good for our body systems.

Anti-Aging Quick Tip: Deep breathing slows the heart rate, regulates blood pressure, dissipates muscle tension, and restores mental and emotional equanimity. (*1001 Ways to Stay Young Naturally*[39])

This emphasis on breathing techniques enhances mind-body integration that teaches us to reconnect with our body so that we can pay attention to what it is saying and make good use of that information. We first looked at this concept back in the very first part, chapter 2 of this book. It is my firm belief that we can never pay too much attention to what our soma is trying to tell us. Our bodies know what is needed, if we will listen more closely and heed the messages being sent. *Grow Younger, Live Longer*[53] echoes that idea to enhance mind-body integration with breathing techniques. *Looking After Your Body: An Owner's Guide to Successful Aging*[56] agrees, and shares some of the practices we can use that focus on our breathing and more:

Relaxation Practices

√   Yoga (integrates mind, body, and spirit)
√   Tai Chi (moving meditation)
√   Qigong (meditation and self-healing)
√   Reiki (transfer of life force from giver to receiver)

Similarly noted in *Your Skin, Younger,*[69] these forms of relaxation and mind-body-spirit integration provide dual benefits for the price of one session because they bring together movement with emotional well-being. **Bonus ROI!**

> ## Anti-Aging Quick Tip: Yoga is one form of exercise and meditation that can be done at any age!

Yoga is my relaxation practice choice. It is a five-thousand-year-old practice that can be undertaken by almost anyone at any time in his/her life (*The Metabolic Plan*[78]). And, as noted in *1001 Ways to Stay Younger*,[39] yoga is an excellent form of exercise for mind and body, being great for stress-busting and energizing. Yoga also is very powerful for balance and posture, which helps prevent falls, one of the significant risks of getting older.

Additionally, WebMD reported that women who do yoga tend to weigh less than others, according to a study in the *Journal of The American Dietetic Association*, probably because yoga regulars use a more "mindful" approach to eating. According to the article "Calming the Fat Away" (*O Magazine*[90]), researchers at UCSF looked at this link between mindfulness and abdominal fat: participants tuned into the physical sensations of hunger, fullness, and taste satisfaction, and learned to eat based on that awareness.

Those with greatest improvement in mindfulness and stress levels lost the largest amount of belly fat. This may be explained, at least in part, by reduction in cortisol levels; under stress, cortisol binds to fat cells, triggering them to store more fat. Another part is that when we become aware of our bodies' "talk" about fullness, we will eat less (website article[22]). So, mindfulness isn't only good for relaxation, but can also help us with how we eat and our weight. Another twofer!

My yoga adventure, which I started almost two years ago now, is a very big part of my PEP program because I find it not only relaxes me, but it helps with stiffness, back pain, or hip pain, or even my sometimes sore, torn cartilage knee. It works my core muscles, which are extremely important to our bodies, and has helped me gain muscle volume, which I would not have guessed to be a consequence when I started. It has improved and made me much more conscious of my posture as well. I stand and walk taller after my one-hour yoga classes twice a week. This is good, very good.

> Yoga is unique in that it addresses the entire person: It exercises and tones the body. It energizes yet soothes the mind. It helps the practitioner achieve a deeply meditative state.

> (Forever Young[71])

According to *Fifty Things to Do When You Turn 50*[91] whether you're a couch potato or a seasoned athlete, yoga can free your body in ways you never dreamed possible. Yoga can:

- Reduce stress and manage both depression and blood pressure.

- Strengthen every muscle in your body.

- Burn calories and manage or lose weight.

- Improve your flexibility and ability to do more in life.

- Promote good posture and decrease back pain.

- Enhance concentration, clarity, and mental focus.

- Improve balance, both on and off the mat.

- Add something fun and joyous to your day.

- Increase your confidence and creativity.

- Help you sleep better and longer.

- **Provide a community of friends.**

I personally have experienced almost all these with yoga, and I highly recommend it to anyone and everyone, no matter his/her age. I talk it up whenever I have someone willing to listen. It definitely works for me, and giving it a try if you can is worth the time and effort. I promise.

In summary, like there is with deep breathing, there are physical benefits to the meditation side of these relaxation practices, such as lowered blood pressure, lowered stress hormones, improved digestion, lowered anxiety, improved sleep and memory, and allowing freshness to emerge, as noted in *Living Longer for Dummies*.[57] They also provide time for us to be alone with ourselves and experience introspection.

> *I think it's very healthy to spend time alone. You need to know how to be alone and not be defined by another person.*
>
> —Oscar Wilde

As an aside, I love Oscar Wilde. I have used a couple of his quotes for all of the thirty years lecturing around the country about periodontics. He really speaks to me (which worries me a little, as he was quite eccentric), but I think his point is very well taken, and I am certain that many/most of us do not spend enough time alone with ourselves. On a final note, here are a few tidbits worth considering on the role and value of solitude and introspection:

Solitude allows us to illuminate what is keeping us from living now the happiest way we can in the circumstances we are in.

(The Gift of Years: Growing Older Gracefully[20])

Silence gives you a chance to be aware of your whole self: body, mind and soul.

(Creative Aging[65])

Self-reflection is necessary throughout life, but even more so as we get older.

(Juicy Living, Juicy Aging[50])

SECTION 2: OUR COCOON

Aging does not happen in isolation or in a vacuum. It happens as a cocktail of things that contribute in both positive and negative ways to our well-being and our aging gracefully pathway. We are impacted by all that we experience, as a result of all the choices we make, including the very surroundings we place the soma in. I think that when we pay attention to that inner voice, we gravitate, or are drawn to, the things that can contribute in a positive way to our well-being, including our environment. For me, it includes things like certain colors, the sound of music all around me, the aesthetics of a beautiful bouquet of flowers, scent, variable intensity and colored lighting, and the look of sunshine through crystals hanging in the windows, to name a few that come right to mind. Here are some other aging expert bits of advice in the area of our cocoon that I came across in my research:

- **Have nothing in your house that is not useful or beautiful.**

(Healthy at 100[14])

- **Create a warm and welcoming feeling in your home, listen to music, surround with art, textures,** comfortable furniture, photos, natural light, and plants.

(The Longevity Bible[42])

I don't believe we think about or consider the impact of our surroundings enough. But I believe strongly that it is worth our while to pay attention to this aspect of our lives. If we think about personally having nothing in our home that is not useful or beautiful, pursuing our next spring cleaning could be quite a significant event, and could result in pretty drastic changes for some of us. That process may also be good for our brain. As I mentioned early in the book, uncluttering our environment can help us think more clearly and function more efficiently. I know for certain that this is true for me. Anytime I need to concentrate but am surrounded by clutter, I have to spruce up my surroundings before I go on, so I am glad to have some rationale for what otherwise might look like irrational compulsive behavior.

Here are some other well-being ideas from an aging expert, including our old friend (as in very old, at five-thousand-plus years) from the last section, yoga:

√ **Exercise**
√ **Laugh**

√ Listen to music
√ Memorize poetry or lyrics
√ Make furry friends
√ Commune with nature
√ Do yoga, get a massage or pedicure
√ Volunteer, as it is associated with well-being, happiness, health, and longevity
√ Cherish the camaraderie of friends and family

(Beautiful Brain, Beautiful You[11])

From this list, music is one that has always been especially "cocooning" for me. From the time I was a young child and my father sat me on his knee with my brother, Bill, and sister, Janice, singing to us and teaching us to sing songs he liked, music has been very positive for me. It can be almost any kind of music (except classical—which, interestingly enough, hypes me up, making relaxation out of the question). Like deep breathing and meditation, there are some very positive physical effects from listening to music we enjoy, such as these noted by *Freedom from Disease*.[87]

Music has many effects on body: It can change pulse rate, circulation, blood pressure, metabolic rate, internal

228

secretions related to metabolic change, muscular energy, respiration rate, gastric motility, electrical conductivity of the skin, papillary dilation, and muscle contraction. It can also alleviate chronic pain and lower the amount of anesthesia needed.

Music has charms to soothe a savage breast; i.e., the power to enchant even the roughest of us. Music to our ears, and all the other aspects of our environment affecting our well-being, truly resonates with me. I have always been aware of and very focused on my surroundings and how they make me feel. I enjoy my senses and the feedback they provide me. I hope you do, too.

I say get comfortable, grab a good book, a glass of red wine or a cup of green tea, or meditate while you enjoy some out-door scenery, or surround yourself with things that make you feel good and are relaxing. Breathe deep and pay attention to your breathing and what it tells you. Sleep well tonight and enjoy how good you feel tomorrow. It is very important to find ways to comfort ourselves in the midst of all the chaos in our world. What works for you?

PART 3:

WHAT IS IT ALL ABOUT?

CHAPTER 1:

OUR POWER, OUR LIGHT

SECTION 1: LIVE LONG AND SEE FAR

Given all that we have learned so far about aging gracefully, a question that begs to be asked (and maybe you have already been asking yourself for a while) is, how long do we want to live? Or, we could put a different twist on it and ask how long do we *need* to live? And if we do desire that long life, what character traits contribute to longevity? How can we, and society around us, make the best of those extra years? How can we capitalize on the wisdom and experience of the aged? This last chapter will provide some food for thought about these questions. We will also look at the role of visioning and goal setting on our aging pathway, plus give some consideration to reinventing ourselves and leaving a legacy. Last, but far, far from least, we will pull it all together at the end of the road for this book.

So, let's say you are envisioning for yourself a long life like I am (or maybe you are merely curious about things like I am), and you want to know more about predicting longevity. You might be interested in an eighty-year landmark study; it determined that the best childhood predictor of longevity was conscientiousness. That is the quality of a prudent, persistent, well-organized person (*The Longevity Project*[12]). This was echoed by WebMD (website link[5]), quoting the same eighty-year study and noting that the researchers found that these conscientious people do more things to protect their health, and that they make choices that lead to stronger relationships and better careers, part of the secret to a long life.

I fit the bill here. I love organization and being organized. I love structure and can be persistent to a fault, which on some occasions might be/has been called stubborn (another darn example of how much like my mother I really am). It has been interesting to me as I write this book to reconfirm with myself that since I was quite young, I have seen myself as living to one hundred. After all this research, I have expanded that view to possibly live some years beyond that (maybe even to our true life potential of 120 years, which I have mentioned a few times), and am comfortable with that idea at least **most** of the time! I have gotten very enthusiastic about what aging looks like today.

I know that some would/do say there's no way they want to live that long, but I wonder, is that because they don't want to live long, or because they subscribe to the aging myth that the "look" of aging is that of their parents or grandparents as they aged? After all I have learned while working on this book, quality longevity is within our grasp and most certainly is worth our reflection, as there is much to be gained with advanced years. We will talk more about these personal and societal benefits of the aged later in this chapter.

Let's go out on a limb together: perhaps we can even live as long as we want/need to in order to accomplish everything we wanted/needed to get done while we were here! Many baby boomers (myself included) want to leave a legacy, leaving the world a better place for having been here. We have work that needs to be checked off before we can check out. Maybe it is all as simple as this: live with as much vim and vigor as possible until your work on the planet is done, then go. Could this be another choice we might have, might make? My late mother-in-law, Polly, believed so, based on her interests in astrology and the afterlife. I think she was on the right track. This would be the ultimate control. I like this thought, and intuitively, I do believe it is possible. I can see myself at around age 110 going to sleep one night and very peacefully never waking up after the last item on my "bucket/to-do" list is done. This is very comforting to me.

I do not fear this, but I have to get my work for this lifetime done first.

> *If we want to, we can learn, grow, love and experience profound happiness in our later years.*
>
> *(The Mature Mind[30])*

The work we need to do could be all about learning the lessons we need to learn. Perhaps Earth is a schoolroom for us all to gain knowledge in, with the ultimate goal to become self-actualized (i.e., self-fulfillment, to actualize your potential). A part of the preplanned, built-in bucket list is to finish our lessons, and we do this via the pathway down which our choices take us. I have a psychic friend who first introduced this concept to me and gave me the name of a great book that elaborates on this topic. It is *Emmanuel's Book: A Manual for Living Comfortably in the Cosmos.* She told me that we are here on this planet, in this and previous and future lifetimes, to learn certain things we need to learn.

Our final "graduation" from this particular school called human incarnation on planet Earth depends on us completing those lessons. When all our lessons are completed, we leave the planet and don't come back in this earthly human form, moving on to a higher form of consciousness. If the lessons are not all learned by the end of the current lifetime, we get to come back and work at it some more in the next lifetime, and so on until we have recognized and made use of our full potential, with all the schoolroom courses checked off.

> **Anti-Aging Quick Tip: Choice, not chance, determines our destiny. Aristotle**

I don't want to go overboard on being spiritual here, but this makes a lot of sense to me, and again my inner voice/gut instinct tells me that it is true. I see our lives on this Earth as part of a grander plan to elevate our consciousness, our awareness. It fits with my belief that everything that happens does so for a reason and not by accident. It would also fit with my view that we are accountable for what happens in our lives (and therefore the lessons we learn) by the choices we make, and that it is all part of a "selfie" preplanned lesson plan we came into this life with. I have loved school and learning since I took my first bus ride to kindergarten, so this schoolroom analogy is very harmonic with me.

If it's true that we have ultimate control over our lives, and our exit from the planet, I wonder if we can do accelerated learning and speed up our schooling, perhaps by living longer and working at making wiser choices. That is a rhetorical question to which I do not have an answer, but it is certainly a thought worth contemplating. I would like the answer to be yes, and my gut tells me this is possible. It makes sense to me within my potpourri of other beliefs.

Let's ponder our ultimate control further and the power behind that control. I strongly believe that we can tap into our native potential to influence how things turn out for us. It is a simple concept woven throughout the various topics covered in this book. That concept, echoed by Aristotle, is that choice, not chance, determines our destiny. By making those choices, we are the architect, the planner, the draftsman of our life. Our life is our design. As Abraham Maslow, who brought the theory of self-actualization into prominence, said, "Every person is, in part, his own project and makes himself." Choice is definitely part of our personal power, and all of us have it and exercise it constantly.

The greatest discovery of all time is that a person can change his future by merely changing his attitude.

—Oprah Winfrey

One of the choices we make along the pathway of our lives and another part of our power is the kind of attitude we adopt toward our life and living. Oprah hones in on the role attitude plays in our power and control. I think she is right on. It is way in synchrony with my book research and the resulting book, my intuitive beliefs, and my lifelong observations. This can most certainly be applied to our aging pathway. We can choose to be very positive about all that comes with longevity, or not. We can see ourselves as aging gracefully and then age gracefully, or not. It is our choice, as it is with all aspects of our life each moment, each day, each year that goes by. Not at all surprisingly, having a positive attitude in general also contributes to longevity.

But, there is more to our power than just choice. Our personal power is as multifaceted as the individual soma (body) and spirit combination. *Super Brain*[94] describes it as including self-confidence, good decision making, trusting gut feelings, being optimistic, having influence over others, having high self-esteem, turning desires into actions, and having the ability to overcome obstacles. There is most certainly a lot of power potential within that list, and the more I consider it, the more expansive and impactful it feels to me, almost Superman-ish in nature. Humans having extraordinary power is what we are talking about here.

We certainly can use our personal power to enhance our longevity. Here is how *The Longevity Bible*[42] summarizes ideas about that, *including* the concept of mastering our environment (via our attitude and the choices we make):

Longevity 8

☐ *Sharpen your mind.*
☐ *Keep a positive outlook.*
☐ *Cultivate healthy relationships.*
☐ *Promote stress-free living.*
☐ *Master your environment.*
☐ *Shape up.*
☐ *Eat for longevity.*
☐ *Get the most out of modern medicine.*

A character trait that I think should be added to any longevity list because it also plays a role in our personal power and control is our creativity, which is driven by our enthusiasm and passion. We can stay youthful in our mind by being creative, acting out of character every so often, and not taking things for granted, which keeps the brain and body acting young and promotes feelings of well-being, which is associated with greater longevity (*1001 Ways to Stay Young Naturally*[39]). *Living Longer for Dummies*[57] offered the following about being creative in elder years:

- Accept the ongoing responsibility to remain creative.

- Believe in your capacity to give something of value that may endure, nurture, teach, comfort.

- Model your effort on those whom you respect.

- Test market your ideas for their potential effectiveness.

- Look for what might be a sure thing.

- Look at the political process for possible creative opportunities.

- Allow yourself to be surprised.

I am actually currently in the process of experiencing the next-to-last idea on that list. Recently, I became a governor-appointed member of the Washington State Council on Aging. I never dreamed that researching and writing this book would lead to being a thought leader/expert at the Governor's Aging Summit last October or that it would further lead to this recent appointment. I am viewing this definitely as a creative learning opportunity for me that I am thrilled about and that is good for me as part of my aging gracefully goal.

Creativity pumps me up. I get excited at any opportunity to fire up my creative juices. It is a wonderful way to express my inner self outwardly, and I enjoy the fruits of my labor with plentiful and intense joy and pride, even if it's as simple as a newly decorated swag on the front door. Creativity is invigorating and it expands our horizons. As said in *Grow Younger, Live Longer*:[53] "By cultivating flexibility and creativity in consciousness, you renew yourself in every moment and reverse the aging process." Yes. I think so.

As I see it, at least part of the fuel for creativity is curiosity. As we have discussed earlier, curiosity is a very powerful motivator and another plus on the score sheet for aging gracefully. *Juicy Living, Juicy Aging*[50] says this: we can use our curiosity to infuse our spirit, keeping us young. To be curious is to wonder, and I do wonder about so many things. There have been very few things in my life that I have not been curious about (accounting comes right to mind on the "not" curious side of the equation). That curiosity and wonder have certainly been very motivating for me, and I don't see that changing as I age. I am every bit as curious now as I have ever been, perhaps even more so because my view of the world is so much more expansive at age sixty-two and a half, because as one of my mentors, Dr. Saul Schluger, used to say: the more I know, the more I **don't** know, and therefore the more there is to wonder about.

As noted in *Retirement Is Not for Sissies*,[37] there is no age limit on wonder and we can stay young by awakening with anticipation, seeing with fascination, and noticing great things first. Every day is a clean slate for us to draw, design, and reinvent ourselves. Every day has new opportunities to learn and grow. How the slate ends up looking is at least in part about attitude coupled with creativity and curiosity. For myself, I know this is true.

Before we move on, let's review the key points so far in this chapter. We can choose to live long; our earthly incarnation is all about learning lessons we need to learn; our attitude is very important and powerful; we have many power tools that give us a lot of control over the shape our life journey takes; being creative and curious, or having wonder, are part of that power and control to age gracefully. Our life is a composition: a unique woven tapestry/painting/sculpture that shows the world who we truly are on the inside. Good. Now let's consider how we can make the best of whatever years we do live.

In the end, it's not the years in your life that count. It's the life in your years.

—Abraham Lincoln

Assuming that the book is still interesting and we are still interested in our longevity and aging gracefully, we might ask, what do we need to think about to make the best of those extra years and really shine in the latter part of our life? *Full Catastrophe Living*[2] put it this way: ***"The real question, and the real adventure, is how do we live our lives while we have the chance?"*** Or, as Jimmy Buffett said, expressing his idea about living, "I'd rather die while I'm living than live while I'm dead," which I interpret to mean he wants to really live it up as he ages versus wasting away...

Our attitude and our choices are the loom or canvas to help us make the best of our years here. They produce that artistic composition of our life that expresses who we are. Our individual tapestry/painting/sculpture can be bright and cheery or in many shades of gray; it is a collage of any, and every, thing we have done. As Dorothy Sander said: "We are all artists. We just create on our own unique kind of canvas." I say, we are all artists and we create our own lives.

> Live your life and forget your age.
>
> —Norman Vincent Peale

Do we want to "live it up" or do want to be part of the living dead? Are we excited about life or bored to tears? Do we want to live long and well, or not? Do we view the common challenges of aging as incentives, rather than hindrances (as proposed in *I Like Being Old*[67])? Incentives are very powerful motivators. They are another fuel to propel us in positive directions, helping us make the best of the years in our lives on planet Earth. Hindrances are de-motivating obstacles to our forward progress. Do we choose forward motion or blocked/stagnant? Is there "movement" in our tapestry or painting, or is it a series of squares and rectangles with thick, defined borders? Is the art piece black, or shades of gray? Or is it deep hues of the colors that speak of vibrancy and "aliveness"?

For myself, I choose forward movement. I want to try to make the very best of the days I have remaining here. I want to graduate from this school called Earth. This reminds me of a related thought. One of my mentors early in my career, a young periodontist, died of heart failure one morning in the shower. She had always told me to live every day as if it were my last, because she knew her life would be short due to a genetic heart defect. Most of us don't know, or don't want to know, about that, but her message has lingered in my mind all these years since she died in 1975. I try to remind myself of that message because, one day at a time, I want to be as fully engaged as I can. I want to have the best life I am capable of while I am still here. Forward motion to make the best of our years is ours to seize. Carpe diem!

Anti-Aging Quick Tip: Embrace creativity regularly to ward off dementia.

During my book research, I read an article based on a **PBS** special (website article[54]) that expands on making the most of our aged years and shares some standards that we might set for ourselves to continue to have a life worth living:

- Take care of your body and your mind will follow; i.e., preserve memory and creativity starting with regular exercise, a healthy diet, and deep sleep.

- Reduce stress through playfulness and meditation (i.e., imagination time can reduce stress).

- Limit the effect of chronic inflammation, and bolster the immune system.

- Embrace creativity regularly—for example, participate in music and dance to ward off dementia, get a museum membership, or take a drawing class (the possibilities are endless).

- Exercise your abilities and learn new skills i.e., true learning—not just solving puzzles.

Those are their suggested keys to hopeful aging.

Deviating slightly from making the most of our aged years, I want to take note that those keys are strikingly representative of many of the major concepts we have been covering in this book. This tells me that the information is on the right track, that it is a good fit in our world. That is very encouraging to me because, as I said a couple of times already in this book, when experts from varying perspectives come to consensus, it has been my experience that what they believe is true.

> The greatest potential for growth and self-realization exists in the second half of life.
>
> —Carl Jung

Back on subject, making the most of our lives is about realizing the full potential that we brought with us into our current lifetime. Longevity breeds developmental opportunity. It is more time to discover our inner self, our inner potential, and more time to make use of that potential. As said in *The Gift of Years: Growing Older Gracefully*,[20] our elder years are for the development of the soul. *The 100 Year Lifestyle*[31] says that it is important to find the energy to change our life and not hold back from change because we think we are too old. Longevity is also about making commitments to be involved with others and to care about something, which gives us a sense of purpose, as noted in *Younger Next Year.*[36] Those longer years extend our road to self-fulfillment/self-actualization. They lead us closer to our ultimate graduation from this schoolroom Earth. They provide us an opportunity to shine out into our world. Why would we ask for anything more?

To have that opportunity to make the most of our lives requires that we get older (which I think is far superior to the alternative). I, for one, feel fortunate to have made it this far. This is very poignant for me, as I lost my two youngest sisters, one in her forties and one in her fifties. They were gone way too soon, but their loss does help remind me of my own good fortune to still be here. From early in this book: "**Do not regret growing older. It is a privilege denied to many.**" Enough said on that, I think the message is very clear.

In youth we learn...in age we understand.

——Marie von Ebner-Eschenbach

Reaping the benefits of longevity is also part of making the best of those extra years to really "shine." And, there are some real tangible benefits to living longer: only age brings wisdom, which is defined as the quality of having experience (and competence), knowledge, and good judgment; the quality of being wise. Wisdom, along with social intelligence {the capacity to effectively negotiate complex social relationships and environments} and memory are the fruits of aging alone (*The Mature Mind*[30]). There is no other way to gain these three things. The ageds achieve the higher grades of the schoolroom Earth. Many lessons learned. Much understanding gained. Many memories stored.

As already noted, the value of aging is much greater than wisdom alone, and as shared in *Healthy Aging*,[29] we can and should discover and realize that value; it adds richness to life, brings maturity, smoothes the "diamond in the rough," and maybe most importantly, develops voice as a living link to the past. We ageds are the reservoir for both personal and societal legacy. We carry the memories. This is irreplaceable perspective and commands respect. The past helps us understand where to go, or maybe as importantly, where *not* to go, in the future. That irreplaceable perspective, coupled with wisdom, competence, and social intelligence, has tremendous contributory worth to our own lives and the world we live in.

In spite of all this, US society seems deficient to me in the area of respect for the ageds and their potential, compared to other societies in the world. Not that this has never been considered in our country. Marc Freedman, in his 1999 book *Prime Time: How Baby Boomers Will Revolutionize Retirement and Transform America*,[24] quoted John F. Kennedy from 1956:

> Today we are wasting resources of incalculable value: the accumulated knowledge, the mature wisdom, the seasoned experience, the skilled capacities, the productivity of a great and growing number of our people—our senior citizens.

Even though that will be more than fifty years ago by the time this book is out, I don't see this as having become an integrated part of the social fabric of our nation. There is awareness about this out there, but it has not moved very far forward toward full functionality. It feels to me like the time has come to get on this bandwagon of respect for the ageds and making use of their potential. Interestingly, one of the most defining features of the cultures known for the health of their elders is a profound respect for the elderly (*Healthy at 100*[14]). *The Metabolic Plan*[78] provides a model of some adjectives that might be used to show that respect:

Hunter-Gatherer (HG) adjectives
for their elders:

☐ Wise
☐ Respected
☐ Venerable (accorded a great deal of respect because of age, wisdom)
☐ Beloved
☐ Experienced

So, let me restate that: our Paleolithic HG ancestral elders were respected, beloved, and attributed with wisdom. One of the most defining features of the cultures known for the health of their elders is profound respect for the elderly (*Healthy at 100*[14]). So, as I understand it, when societal views value the aged, it plays a positive role in their health and well-being, which allows them to reach more of their potential, making them subsequently greater contributors to their society. Positive breeds positive; it is a reinforcing cycle. And from the same aging expert: "How we treat ourselves and each other always matters." Yes, it does. Respect is key.

Looking for some positives about how US society views our aged, I did discover that there are some programs out there for us aged to give back and to be respected, valued contributors. Freedman[24] lists some of them: Foster Grandparent Program, Senior Companion Program, Hilton Head Volunteers, Civic Ventures, Experience Corps/Vista, Princeton Project 55, National Senior Service Corps, Peace Corps, Score (Service Corps of Retired Executives), America's Promise, etc. That is a start, but I think it woefully undercreates the opportunities for the boomer age wave that is beginning now. We need to keep beating this drum and hitting this concept home until it truly becomes part of our social norm. Our society needs to capitalize on JFK's "resources of incalculable value"—i.e., the aged as they realize their full potential.

With the magnitude of the boomer generation, the potential that is coming down the pike right now has never been seen. The sometimes called "silver tsunami" is full of incredible power, with potential widespread impact in many different places in our society. Why not use some of that tremendous wealth of wisdom, memory, and competence to influence our magnificent country in a very positive direction, all the while reversing the aging process and improving the longevity of the aged in that age wave so they can continue to contribute, which improves their longevity so they can continue to contribute, and so on?

It is good for us aged personally, and it creates the opportunity for our legacies, allowing us to self-actualize while making our world a better place! In the political arena alone, think of the potential we have to change the way things are done, as many of us wished we had been able to do when we were young protestors! Freedman[24] offers his view and some strategies on how we might take advantage of the age wave:

Four strategies to take us in the right direction:

- **Develop a new vision for a new age (of the contributions that older Americans might make to American life).**

- **Build the breakthrough institution (targeted to lifelong learning, new opportunities to contribute, the chance to promote health and well-being both physical and spiritual, a community of like-minded individuals, and a place to help navigate the passage to this new stage of life).**

- **Create good places to grow older; i.e., communities that think more systematically, comprehensively and strategically about how they might make the most of the aging society.**

- **Launch a "Third-Age Bill"; e.g., a bill to ease the relicensing of retired volunteer physicians.**

Paul Irving, CEO of the Milken Institute, put another spin on the age wave potential: "Economic growth occurs at the intersection of demography and innovation." That intersection is already here. Why not take advantage? Why not make the best that we can of the boomer age wave? Why not let the "silver tsunami" fuel our forward progress to enhance our world economically?

Having just participated in Washington State Governor Jay Inslee's Aging Summit and being a new governor-appointed member of the Washington State Council on Aging, I have had several conversations about the age wave potential in the last six to eight months. It is clear that ageds bring a lot to the table, and I think our society could make great use of this unprecedented, powerful resource that has already started rolling in. It is a win-win. We only lose if we don't pursue it. Enough said about that. Respectfully, we can move on now to talk about goals and visioning.

SHOW ME THE WAY

If we do want to live long and healthy, and if we are open to being accountable for ourselves by the choices we make, and if we are receptive to learning the lessons we came here to learn and making the best of our years on planet Earth, how do we go about that? How do we figure out the right path to take? One aging authority offers this advice:

> *Look inward to your likes and dislikes. You will find things in your life that are part of your nature and things that go against it. Create a life that is congruent with your attitudes and beliefs.*
>
> *(Bill Frank's Forever Young[45])*

In other words, we can *let our inner voice* give us direction for our path forward. That inner voice can help us set and achieve our goals. This is important because goal setting is another determinant of our aging gracefully pathway. That is how I came to write this book. One of my former hygiene staff persons gave me a book at my big sixtieth birthday and retirement party.

There was an exercise in the book that had me write down what I would like to accomplish in the next five years. I found myself writing down that I wanted to research and author a book on aging. I could see myself writing that book. It was a goal I could very clearly envision, and I knew in my gut that it was the right direction for me. Visioning is a key here. As was said in *Old Is the New Young*,[58] we need to have goals and a vision for our lives. We cannot get to where we want to be if we can't envision the destination we are trying to reach. As I said in the very first chapter of this book, *"You can't get somewhere unless you know where it is that you are trying to go."* I have lived my entire life using this personal credo, and I am absolutely convinced that it is a universal doctrine that we can all make use of. We will come back to visioning in a moment.

A necessary part of visioning and goal setting is about trusting our gut feelings. The value of these intuitive thoughts is way underestimated and too often ignored, in my opinion. As we talked about earlier from *Super Brain*,[94] part of our personal power is about trusting our gut feelings. Many years back, shortly after I started my periodontal practice, I read an article about the top CEOs and what they had in common. Interestingly, all those top CEOs said that they made important business decisions based on both facts and their intuition.

That finding was profound and very personally reinforcing for me as a new businessperson. I have since come to firmly believe that although facts are helpful, the ultimate "best" decision needs to be based on what intuitively feels right. My intuition always leads me in the right direction. It has always made me aware of the doors that were open for me to step through. Try it. I think you will like it. Goal setting based on trusting our intuitive selves—an essential, very powerful, and effective combination to design the path of our aging journey. Let's talk more now about being able to envision our goals and the role it plays in achieving them.

Anti-Aging Quick Tip: Envision it, and it shall come.

If you haven't read Richard Bach's *Illusions,* it is a short, simple book that is well worth the time spent. There's an exercise in it about imagining an object, like a blue feather, then focusing on thoughts that envision that object. I did that exercise way back in the late '80s, focusing on picturing the blue feather in my mind for a week or two a couple of times each day, until one day I simply forgot about it. Many months later, I was helping my sister, Janice, move, and as I was vacuuming, I saw something blue in the carpet—yes, it was the blue feather! At first, I could not believe I was actually seeing and picking up a blue feather, as I had envisioned. Could it be true that envisioning something could bring that something into our reality? Could it really be that simple? I was awestruck by this and have never forgotten it or the lesson it teaches: envision it and it will come. Envisioning and goal setting based on our intuition are two more aspects of the innate power and control we have over what happens in our lives. I try not to either underuse or underestimate either one of them.

SECTION 2: REINVENT AND LEGACY

SPARKLE AND SHINE

Reinvent yourself: Shift your gaze forward. Recognize your strengths and look beyond your limitations. Find new activities and attitudes to replace ones that no longer work.

(I Like Being Old: A Guide to Making the Most of Aging[67])

As we have been discussing, a long, quality life is an opportunity to realize our full potential by visioning and goal setting where we want to go and where we want to end up. Reinventing ourselves is one possible outcome. Last summer, I wrote and published a web article titled "Live Long and Legacy" that expresses some thoughts about reinventing ourselves. I see it as another important piece of the aging gracefully puzzle. Reinventing ourselves is a process of change that allows us to expose our inner light and cast it forward into the world. That inner light encompasses enthusiasm, creativity, and being inspirational. It is having awareness, humor, compassion, and flexibility.

I shared thoughts that reinvention has a lot of creative potential, and that being creative in our endeavors has a built-in, intrinsic reward that allows us to renew, restart, and recommence ourselves. We have already talked about creativity as a big piece of the aging gracefully mosaic. Do we see the challenges in our lives as "sparkling moments" to change, experiment, push ourselves, and grow (*Forytude*[17])? Do we aspire to "joie de vivre," as noted in The *Mature Mind*[30]? Do we relate to this quote from *Unexpectedly Eighty*:[38] "I don't intend to fade away. There's still a tune or two I'd like to play"? Have we ever shared this thought from Chili Davis?

Growing old is mandatory; growing up is optional.

All that having been said, I do not underestimate the effort and courage needed to reinvent ourselves. It is scary. It is a leap of faith with no literal or absolute guarantee about where we will land. It instills fear in us, but faith pushes us over the edge to fly. The PBS special that I mentioned earlier in this chapter says this about reinventing ourselves: "As we age, we gain insight, vision and wisdom, all of which serve our creativity well, if we just work up the courage to jump in and try once again to see the world anew" (website article[54]). Yes, it takes courage, no question about that, but let's do it. **Let's roll!**

Some talk about reinventing ourselves as something we do after retirement. But could it better be viewed as the *alternative* to retirement? I got started on this line of thinking after a phone conversation with Milken Institute CEO Paul Irving, during which he said that the word *retirement* should be retired. That struck a chord with me, because when I sold my practice two years ago, I had told people that I was not retiring but reinventing myself. Since then, though, I hadn't given any thought to the difference in meaning between those two words until Paul mentioned it.

The word *retirement* means ending, withdrawal, ceasing to work. *Retire* does not fit. Wrong word. Wrong meaning. Wrong implication. Wrong destiny. Wrong period for us boomers and beyond. No rocking chair on the porch for the boomers! *Prime Time: How Baby Boomers Will Revolutionize Retirement and Transform America*[24] said that the boomers will refuse to be taken out of circulation; that they would retread instead of retire. So we could assign the moniker retreadment to replace retirement!

Or, I have another idea: I suggest that we replace retirement with reinventment.

Let's pursue defining this new term. Reinventment would be the stage of our lives when we leave our major career work and begin the work of redesigning ourselves to maximize all of our potential, our inner light, our soul—i.e., who we really are. It is *leaving the path we've been on to head in a new direction and finish what we came here for, as contrasted to retirement, which is an act of ending or withdrawal from an active working life.*

Reinventment certainly more accurately describes what I think of when I ponder my journey after leaving my thirty-plus-year primary career as a gum surgeon. I became an author and an aging expert/thought leader. I have redesigned myself. I am reinvented, not retired or retreaded. I really identify with the concept presented by the aging expert from thirty-plus years ago that the boomers will work until they die. We are all about reinventment. I know I am because I have trouble sitting still.

That reminds me of a conversation I had with my mother one time, where she pointed out to me that even on vacation I keep constantly busy doing "stuff." I replied that "that is just the nature of this beast," and it is. I can't see myself, or boomers in general, stopping and sitting around quietly without a "bucket/ to-do" list. I see us being active right up to check-out time, continuing to contribute in our world and living longer than any prior generation. "Some form of meaningful work is part of the rhythm of life" (*Retirement Is Not for Sissies*[37]). No retirement there, just reinventment.

Newly found success and an ensuing legacy can be an important part of reinventment. Success is not only for the young, as many successful legacies have been created by societal elders. How do we define a successful legacy? I personally am confident that it is not defined by either monetary or material wealth, except in the context of how those might be used to contribute to the greater good. Bill and Melinda Gates come to mind here. Another way to think about legacy is living out our purpose(s) in life. The aging book *The Gift of Years: Growing Older Gracefully*[20] noted: "In our dreams lies our unfinished work for the world." In our dreams lies our reinventment and completion of the to-do list we came into this world with. In our dreams lies the work of finishing this life's lessons. Those dreams are the precursor to our legacy.

Anti-Aging Quick Tip: Live Long and Legacy!

Certainly we boomers believe in leaving a legacy, as noted by numerous sources, including *The Big* Shift.[27] This is the baby boomers' clarion call, just as the aging expert from the late '80s, which I spoke about in the beginning of this book, had said. Our generation does not plan to sit back and sit still for the rest of our time on this planet after we leave the nine-to-five traditional work world. Oh no! We are boomers! We will never actually retire; we will reinvent ourselves and find a new direction to plug our energy into as we strive to expose our inner light and cast it forward in the world as our legacies.

> *What counts in life is not the mere fact that we have lived. It is what difference we have made to the lives of others that will determine the significance of the life we lead.*
>
> —Nelson Mandela

As noted earlier, we have a lot of potential to make an impact on our world in many positive ways. We are a BIG group with lots of BIG ideas and aspirations. This kind of inner drive to leave a legacy is another big piece of the aging gracefully puzzle. And guess what? As I said earlier in this chapter, when we live longer, we have more opportunity to define our purpose and to leave our legacies (I quote myself here): "Longevity breeds developmental opportunity. It is more time to discover our inner self/ soul, our inner potential and, more time to make use of that potential." Legacy is about commitment and having a sense of purpose to our lives.

The great use of life is to spend it for something that will outlast us.

—William James, The 100 Year Lifestyle[31]

As I write about legacy, I am getting up close and personal with myself about it: What legacy have I left so far, and what else still needs to be done? I ask myself, have I lived up to Leo Rosten's view of this? He said: ***"The purpose of life is to matter—to count, to stand for something, to have it make some difference that we lived at all."*** Well, I have taught graduate students about being an excellent periodontist, and I have lectured to my colleagues about excellence in periodontal surgery and have published ten scientific papers, so there is some legacy there. Periodontal practice was an awesome thirty-year ride during which I had the legacy pleasure to help people get their gum tissue healthy and keep their teeth, but I hope this book will be my most impactful legacy so far by contributing to my fellow humans being able to live longer, healthier lives and by shedding some light on respecting that part of our society that carries the society's wisdom and societal memory: You got it! They got it! We got it! **Us aged!**

Will there be more legacy for me after this book? I have a second book in mind, and certainly I am confident that there is still more unfinished work in my dreams to become reality. I simply have to envision and set goals and then listen to my inner voice to blast forward on the leap of faith, without restriction or regret!

A man [or woman] is not old until regrets take the place of dreams.

—John Barrymore

Speaking of regret, which is another attitudinal choice, it need not be part of the picture on our aging gracefully pathway. The past was the past that was needed to bring us to where we are now, so that we can be comfortable with who we are moving forward, not mourning who we are not. Regret is energy that might otherwise be used to propel us onto a very positive path, helping us to discover our full potential.

Nothing is IMPOSSIBLE, the word itself says, I'M POSSIBLE!

—Audrey Hepburn

There is nothing we can't do, if we make up our minds to do it, and don't get in our own way, in my opinion. Reinventing ourselves and being creative also requires that we not restrict ourselves by arguing for our limitations, because if we do, it is certain that they will be ours to keep—and that simply has way too much dimming effect. That thought is my slightly revised version of one of my favorite quotes:

> *Argue for your limitations, and sure enough, they're yours.*
>
> —*Richard Bach*

SECTION 3: MIRROR IMAGE TWO: UNTIL WE MEET AGAIN

THE END OF THE ROAD, FOR NOW

Well, this book as been quite a journey. We have studied the aging battlefield and have defined the troops and weaponry available to help us win the war. We have taken a journey inward to our soul and personal power. We have replaced the word retirement with a new moniker, reinventment. We have talked about legacy as the manifestation of our dreams. I hope you have gotten as much useful, everyday information out of reading it as I have doing the research and writing it.

I have reinvented myself as an author now, and that inspires me. I am excited to share what I have learned, hoping it will make a real difference in my fellow and future ageds' lives. As a reminder, this work is information I selected as important to the aging concept but *through my filters, biases, and lenses.* I concur with Victor Hugo when he said: "We do not claim that the portrait we are making is the whole truth, only that it is a resemblance." This book is my resemblance of the truth about aging based upon what aging experts have shared and how I have perceived their messages.

Man's mind once stretched to a new idea never goes back to its original dimensions.

—Oliver Wendell Holmes, Sr.

For certain, my mind has been permanently stretched in a very positive, new direction for having looked at and bundled all this information into a book. I have used and still am using it to change my own choices, one tidbit at a time. I like the physical benefits of aging gracefully. Most days, I like what I see in the mirror now: better posture, nicely shaped legs, a waist of thirty-one to thirty-two inches, a fairly symmetrical hourglass shape, a face with vibrancy and with which I strive to smile more. My balance is improved, as is my flexibility and strength. My weight is holding fairly steady at 141–144 pounds. My joints hurt less, I have more energy. I wish all these things, and many, many more, for all of you!

Like I did as a periodontist with my patients, it is one step at a time, with constant reevaluations to ascertain progress and determine the next steps. Nothing is etched in concrete; our aging pathway is a constantly evolving, morphing sculpture, tapestry, painting, or whatever piece of art best portrays who we are. We are the architect and artist of our life, and I believe that we came into this world equipped with all the right paintbrushes, looms, or sculpting tools to have complete control over how it turns out.

And, as I have said many times in this book, I believe that we are each accountable for where we are at any moment in our lives as a result of the choices we make each moment, each day, each year. As stated in *The Aging Myth*,[34] how well we age will be highly influenced by our lifestyle choices such as good sleep, brain stimulation, a healthy diet, regular exercise, watching our sugar intake, etc., and excellence in our personal health is never an accident. Aristotle echoes that in his very well-said piece on excellence:

Excellence is never an accident. It is always the result of high intention, sincere effort, and intelligent execution; it represents the wise choice of many alternatives—choice, not chance, determines your destiny.

So, my journey is in full gear now. As I am finishing writing this book, I am now sixty-two and a half years old. I am still incorporating many of these bits of expert advice on aging into my life and lifestyle and I am honestly enjoying it! It is important to remember, though, that progress check-ins are important, as are remaining open to new, additional ideas and concepts, listening carefully to our inner voice, and recognizing that there is always room for improvement. Remember, too, that 80 percent effort yields 95 percent benefit. We have some leeway to be perfectly imperfectly human while striving for excellent. NOTE: I did not say perfection. I don't believe in striving for perfection, but rather in striving for excellent.

We also need to remember to reward ourselves for our successes and set new goals for our desired and envisioned destination. We can capitalize on the power of our intuition and envisioning to achieve our goals. We can work on the legacies we want to leave. There will be steps forward and some back. There will be good days and days that are not so good. We have to have acceptance but not regret when we relapse at times into old, bad choices. Things will be as they should be along the way. Our challenge is to recognize these poor choices and replace them with other choices that serve us better, without arguing for our own limitations. Another important thing is to savor our lives—savor the moment, savor the information our senses take in, savor our very existence—savor, period. I hope at the end that we will skid in sideways, used up, totally worn out, and screaming, "Woo-hoo, what a ride! I also hope we might share this thought from Erma Bombeck:

> *When I stand before God [higher power] at the end of my life, I would hope that I would not have a single bit of talent left, and I could say, "I used everything you gave me."*

CHAPTER 2:

PULLING US ALL TOGETHER AND EPILOGUE

I'd rather die while I'm living than live while I'm dead.

—Jimmy Buffett, "Growing Older But Not Up"

We have reached the end of this journey. It is shortly after the holidays and I will begin the process of publication. As per my usual, I have a few extra holiday pounds to get rid of, but I accept that as part of being perfectly imperfectly human. I know and respect the importance of keeping track of what is happening to my body and I hope you do as well. I hope we all will respect the importance of being guided to move forward with appreciation for the magnificent equipment the body is, listening to what it has to say, and acting as its steward to be as good as it can be. We *are* the keeper of the vessel that houses the being.

I said it was the end of the road for what I had to share in the last section. Well, it was the end of the book writing, but I have one last thing I want to do. When I first began this book, my goal was to provide as many tidbits as I possibly could, formatted into bullet points, quotes, text boxes, and lists. I have saved this place in my book to share the ones that I have not yet shared in the book text.

There will be no more of my verbiage after this. From this point on, it will simply be aging expert tidbits, mainly on the general subject of aging gracefully, with some short quips and quotes mixed in. Remember, use what strikes a chord with you and can be incorporated into your life. It is meant to be both practical and biologically sound advice. When it comes to really almost any subject, including this one, all too often I think we reinvent the wheel. In the case of graceful aging, we don't need to. There are some impressive sets of data out there (which follow) about what those who have longevity have in common, so that we can benefit by studying what they have already found out. At least some of it is easy... Some one-hundred-plus authorities later, here are the final tidbits.

*To be forever young: Think young in mind,
be young in body, and feel a spirit at all
times to remain forever young.*

(Bill Frank's Forever Young[45])

10 Steps to Reverse Aging

1. *Change your perceptions.*
2. *Through two kinds of deep rest: restful awareness and restful sleep.*
3. *Nurture your body through healthy food.*
4. *Use nutritional complements wisely.*
5. *Enhance mind/body integration.*
6. *Through exercise.*
7. *Eliminate toxins from your life.*
8. *Cultivate flexibility and creativity.*
9. *Through love.*
10. *Maintain a youthful mind.*

(Grow Younger, Live Longer[53])

"I'm convinced that what we really need most to sustain us we grow older, more than any drug on the market, is this kind of appreciative awareness, along with compassion, a sense of humor, and simple common sense. Side effects will include a certain amount of pain, a fair share of sorrow, recurring doses of discomfort great and small, and an immeasurable, priceless quantity of peace of mind."

(Forward From Here[60])

"The whole of science is nothing more than a refinement of everyday thinking."
Albert Einstein (Live Stronger, Live Longer) 84

Jane Fonda's Ingredients for Successful Aging:

- ☐ Not abusing alcohol.
- ☐ Not smoking.
- ☐ Getting enough sleep.
- ☐ Being physically active.
- ☐ Eating a healthy diet.
- ☐ Maintaining a healthy, active brain through learning.
- ☐ Positivity: Encouraging a positive attitude.
- ☐ Reviewing and reflecting on your life.
- ☐ Loving and staying connected.
- ☐ Generativity: Giving of oneself.
- ☐ Caring about the bigger picture.

(Prime Time[85])

From Full Catastrophe Living: "Certain attitudes and ways of seeing ourselves and others are health-enhancing, that affiliate trust and seeing the basic goodness in others and ourselves has intrinsic healing power; each one of us has an important role to play in our own well-being." (Full Catastrophe Living[2])

"You can't turn back the clock. But you can wind it up again."

Bonnie Prudden

Longevity Steps

- *Laugh often.*
- *Cry when needed. Be humbled by the universe.*
- *Celebrate transitions.*
- *Take pleasure in small things.*
- *Know how much is enough.*
- *Have nothing in your house that is not useful or beautiful.*
- *Consider what you would do if only 6 months to live.*
- *Have affirmations, use visualization.*

- *Be and appreciate what you can be.*
- *Stand for your vision.*
- *Sing, even if you can't sing.*
- *Never be ashamed.*
- *Get enough sleep.*
- *Take time to meditate.*
- *Give thanks.*
- *Respect all life.*
- *Pet cats, dogs, other animals.*
- *Celebrate death days and birthdays.*
- *Celebrate your uniqueness.*
- *Give yourself permission to be healthy, happy and at peace.*

(Healthy at 100[14])

Old is the New Young Secrets:

Secret #1: It *can* be done; i.e., use common sense and a few small investments in your body, mind, social network, and finances.

Secret #2: Think positively.

Secret #3: Care for yourself. There is info everywhere: magazines, books, Internet, TV.

Secret #4: Find your own (health care) team.

Secret #5: Know your weak spots (and work on strengthening them)

Secret #6: Stay curious.

Secret #7: Sharpen your mind.

Secret #8: Build your resilience so you can adjust easily to change, roll with life's punches.

Secret #9: Seek help (don't expect to do everything yourself).

Secret #10: Put your money where it counts.

(Old Is the New Young[58])

The "young old" indicate something entirely new in the offing.

(The Big Shift[27])

Skills Needed to Endure

1. *Redefine health, sex and happiness.*
2. *Get educated about weight loss and aging.*
3. *Stop eating all factory-produced food.*
4. *Eat a balanced diet of real, whole, living food.*
5. *Properly care for and feed your brain.*
6. *Quit addictions.*
7. *Supplement your diet.*
8. *Live a detox lifestyle and flush, rinse, nourish.*
9. *Use HRT if needed.*
10. *Sleep 8 hours.*
11. *Practice self-compassion meditation.*
12. *Exercise regularly.*

(Healthy, Sexy, Happy[28])

C-o-o-l!

- *Cool is ageless, modern, youthful.*
- *Look for "trickle down" styles – high fashion that has been copied or restyled by less expensive clothing and accessories.*
- *The art of the mix: mix pieces of fashion from a past style with something classic.*
- *"If you keep your age and physique in mind you can have great success (and fun) borrowing from the younger generation's style."*
- *An active life provides opportunities for a youthful, sporty style*
- *"Dressing casually is not a license for sloppiness or bad taste."*
- *"Natural fibers and unexpected color combine for creative style."*
- *A current hairstyle and minimal makeup lets your loveliness shine through.*

(Forever Cool[70])

From Juicy Living, Juicy Aging:[50]
Invigorate your vocabulary by adding
some juicy words daily, like "brilliant,"
"luscious," "succulent," "daring,"
"dazzling," and "magnificent."

Centenarian Power: Check!

The number of centenarians increases 8%
per year in the US contrasted to overall
pop. growth of 1%.

Centenarian characteristics:

√ Orderly
√ Industrious
√ Mobile
√ Nonsmoker
√ Frugal
√ Optimistic
√ Patriotic
√ Frisky

√ Religious
√ Curious

(Living Longer for Dummies[57])

Advice: Dine well, stay fit, keep laughing, and enjoy life and the people you share it with.

(Age Proof Your Body[47])

Age Graceful Recipe

☐ Prevention.
☐ Anti-inflammatory diet.
☐ Supplements.
☐ Physical activity.
☐ Rest and sleep.
☐ Touch and sex.
☐ Practice stress reduction.
☐ Maintain social connections.

❏ Be flexible in mind and body.

❏ Discover benefits of aging.

❏ Don't deny reality of aging.

❏ Keep record of lessons you learn, wisdom you gain and values you hold then share it with those you care about. (*Healthy Aging*[29])

8 Proven Keys to a Long, Healthy Life

1. *Exercise your brain to maintain mental vitality.*

2. *Be connected: a sense of belonging also keeps us healthy.*

3. *Get a good night's sleep.*

4. *Get your stress under control.*

5. *Make meaningful contact, have a sense of community.*

6. *Keep up regular physical activity.*

7. *Eat your way into feeling and looking younger.*

8. *Practice prevention: take an active role in managing your health.*

(The Longevity Prescription[1])

Principles to Help You Live Longer to Help You Live Longer

- *Decide to be happy (laughter and smiling are directly related to better health).*
- *Exercise naturally (keep you body flexible and mobile; i.e., HG).*
- *Eat a wide spectrum of foods (not excessive consumption and portion control).*
- *Bond with people (humans are not genetically coded to be hermits).*
- *Rise and shine (i.e., acclimate to the sun).*

- Read (the mind is a terrible thing to waste).
- Learn to love, forgive, and let things go (if something eats at you, it will consume you).
- Manage stress.
- Keep busy.

(The Aging Myth[34])

Lessons Learned from 85 and Beyond

1. Continue to do what you did; i.e., have regular routines that are invested with meaning.
2. Design your living space; i.e., to enable exercise, comfort, a healthy diet, self-care, and avert falls.
3. Live in moderation; i.e., exercise restraint.
4. Take time for self; i.e., experience solitary activities that enable personal growth.

5. *Ask for help; mobilize resources; i.e., negotiate a careful balance between autonomy and dependence.*
6. *Connect with peers; i.e., homogenous peer networks can be socially, physically, and emotionally beneficial.*
7. *Resort to "tomfoolery"; i.e., make fun of yourself and others, use humor.*
8. *Care for others; i.e., care work provides a sense of social and civic belonging.*
9. *Reach out to family; i.e., nobody can do it alone.*
10. *Get intergenerational experience; redefine family; i.e., age-based diversity and community in housing, public spaces, and classrooms.*

11. *Insist on hugs; i.e., reach out to give and receive physical affection.*
12. *Be adaptable; i.e., grow and learn in the context of new challenges.*
13. *Accept and prepare for death; i.e., achieve a personal level of continuity in death.*

(Lessons for Living from 85 and Beyond[73])

4 Long Life Principles

1. *Envision being a happy, healthy 100.*
2. *Design your life to reinforce your goals.*
3. *Diversify most domains of life.*
4. *Invest in science.*

(A Long Bright Future[49])

"My time is valuable, too valuable not to capture every moment I can" N. Hadler

(Rethinking Aging[13])

50 Secrets of Those Who Live Long

- *Eat to 80 percent full.*
- *Eat 5–7 fresh fruits and veggies a day.*
- *Choose buckwheat, brown rice or other whole grains.*
- *Eat sprouted wheat bread.*
- *Use hemp.*
- *Eat meat as a treat.*
- *Prepare your meal right (grill versus fry, chicken over lamb).*
- *Choose organic goat and sheep cheese.*
- *Be full of beans.*
- *Have a good egg.*
- *Find good fats in fish.*
- *Have a handful of nuts and seeds daily.*

- Choose olive oil.
- Beware of fats in disguise (fish and olive oil versus killing fats like poly unsaturated cooking oils).
- Use garlic and onion.
- Discover the power of crunchy veggies.
- Keep aging away with a salad a day.
- Eat sweet potatoes.
- Enjoy pizza without guilt (because of tomatoes and lycopene).
- Snack on apricots.
- Find long life in berries.
- Have yogurt.
- Eat fermented foods (like yogurt, sauerkraut, aged cheese, beer, wine).
- Choose soy.
- Sprout superfoods (beans and seeds).
- Eat mushrooms.
- Remember your herbs.
- Don't pass the salt.
- Chew.

- *Go organic.*
- *Beware the pastry counter.*
- *Red wine with dinner.*
- *Make time for green tea.*
- *Drink water.*
- *Combine your foods (e.g., protein with nonstarchy veggies).*
- *Use juices and saunas to detoxify (i.e.; fast with water or juice, sweating).*
- *Supplement.*
- *Exercise.*
- *Daily sunshine.*
- *Jog your memory.*
- *Breathe and hum.*
- *Sit still and do nothing.*
- *Have faith.*
- *Laugh it off.*
- *Sing in the shower.*
- *Give help to others.*
- *Marry and/or get a dog.*
- *Invite a friend.*
- *Avoid the Standard American Diet (SAD); i.e., meat, dairy, sugar, salt, refined carbohydrates.*

- *Sleep.*

(50 Secrets of the World's Longest Living People[48])

Author's Note: There is some disagreement about how much meat to eat. I tend to agree with the hunter-gatherer concept but the reader should decide how you feel.

Younger, Thinner You:
10 Commandments

1. *Upgrade every meal with spices.*
2. *Drink tea with every meal.*
3. *Eat yogurt daily.*
4. *Choose proteins carefully.*
5. *Choose expanding and balanced foods for weight loss and longevity.*
6. *Eat fiber-filled foods daily.*
7. *Drink water throughout the day.*
8. *Eat color in every meal.*

9. *Eat fruits and veggies both raw and cooked.*
10. *Choose three foods for each meal.*

(Younger [Thinner] You Diet[33])

Longevity 8

☐ Sharpen your mind.

☐ Keep a positive outlook.

☐ Cultivate healthy relationships.

☐ Promote stress-free living.

☐ Master your environment.

☐ Shape up.

☐ Eat for longevity.

☐ Get the most out of modern medicine.

(The Longevity Bible[42])

10 Powerful Longevity Lessons:

1. *Move naturally (i.e., regular, low-intensity physical activity: garden, walk, take the stairs, ride a bike, rake yard, sweep, shovel snow, take yoga).*
2. *Stop eating when your stomach is 80% full (hara hachi bu, which leads to about 1900–2000 calories) and eat slower, earlier.*
3. *Avoid or minimize meat and processed foods (eat nuts, drink lots of water).*
4. *Drink red wine in moderation.*
5. *Have a strong sense of purpose (plan de vida).*
6. *Feel needed.*
7. *Give something back.*
8. *Meditate (take time to relieve stress).*
9. *Participate in a spiritual community; i.e., have faith, make family a priority, have social*

*connectedness with others who
share blue zone values.*
10.*Savor what you have, respect the
elders.*

(Blue Zones[23])

*"The aging process has you firmly in its
grasp if you never get the urge to throw a
snowball."*

D. Larson

*G. Burns at age 95 refused to sign a five-
year contract with Caesar's Palace, saying
he couldn't be sure it would still be there
in five years.*

(The Complete Geezer Guidebook[62])

Economist John Stoven: "Our conception of what qualifies as "old" has become old-fashioned."

(The Big Shift [27])

Vitality Tips and Tricks

Be a lifelong learner.
Think positive.
Volunteer.
Embrace your beliefs.
Rely on pet power.
(Looking After Your Body: An Owner's Guide to Successful Aging [56])

APPENDIX: WEBSITE LINKS

1. https://www.livestrong.com/register/

2. http://www.projectweightloss.com/index.php

3. http://www.realage.com/

4. http://www.bbhq.com/

5. http://www.webmd.com

6. http://home.fuse.net/clymer/bmi/

7. http://pathmed.com/

8. http://www.skin-care.becomegorgeous.com/perfect_skin/prevent_wrinkles_with_face_massage-986.html

9. http://www.prevention.com/health/

10. http://www.nia.nih.gov/health/featured/healthy-aging-longevity

11. http://www.steam-sauna-benefits.com/steam-room-skin-care.html

12. http://www.lifescript.com/Health/Alternative-Therapies/Supplements/The_Benefits_Of_Castor_Oil.aspx

13. http://www.topantiagingtips.com/index.html

14. http://braingym.org

15. http://d22haa4wr85g1q.cloudfront.net/wp-content/uploads/2009/06/brain_quiz.pdf

16. http://www.linesofbeauty.com/2012/10/success-or-pleasure.html?utm_source=feedburner&utm_medium=email&utm_campaign=Feed%3A+LinesOfBeauty+%28Lines+of+Beauty%29

17. http://www.livingto100.com/

18. http://FoodForTheBrain.org

BOOK TABLE OF AUTHORITIES

1. Butler, Robert N. *The Longevity Prescription: The 8 Proven Keys to a Long, Healthy Life.* New York: The Penguin Group, 2010.

2. Kabat-Zinn, Jon. *Full Catastrophe Living.* New York: Bantam Dell, 1990.

3. Friedan, Betty. *The Fountain of Age.* New York: Simon & Schuster, 1993.

4. Forberg, Cheryl. *Prevention Positively Ageless.* New York: Rodale, 2008.

5. Roizen, Michael, and Mehmet Oz. *You Staying Young: The Owner's Manual for Extending Your Warranty.* New York: Free Press, 2007.

6. Kelder, Peter. *Ancient Secret of the Fountain of Youth.* New York: Doubleday Dell Publishing Inc., 1999.

7. Brownstein, David, and Sheryl Shenefelt. *The Guide to Healthy Eating.* Birmingham, Michigan: Publisher Name, 2007.

8. Cooper, Robert K., and Leslie L. Cooper. *Low-Fat Living: Turn off the Fat-Makers, Turn on the Fat-Burners for Longevity, Energy, Weight Loss,_Freedom from Disease.* Emmaus, Pennsylvania: Rodale Press, 1996.

9. Kurzwell, Ray, and Terry Grossman. *Transcend: Nine Steps to Living Well Forever.* New York: Rodale Press, 2009.

10. Grey, Aubrey, and Michael Rae. *Ending Aging: The Rejuvenation Breakthrough That Could Reverse Human Aging in Our Lifetime.* New York: St Martin's Press, 2007.

11. Pasinski, Marie, and Jodie Gould. *Beautiful Brain, Beautiful You: Look Radiant from the Inside Out by Empowering Your Mind.* New York: Hyperion, 2011.

12. Friedman, Howard, and Leslie Martin. *The Longevity Project: Surprising Discoveries for Health and Long Life from the Landmark Eight-Decade Study.* New York: Hudson Street Press, 2011.

13. Hadler, Nortin. *Rethinking Aging: Growing Old and Living Well in an Overtreated Society.* Chapel Hill, North Carolina: University of North Carolina Press, 2011.

14. Robbins, John. *Healthy at 100: The Scientifically Proven Secrets of the World's Healthiest and Longest-Lived Peoples.* New York: Random House, 2006.

15. Wolf, Robb. *The Paleo Solution: The Original Human Diet.* Las Vegas, Nevada: Victory Belt Publishing, 2010.

16. Agronin, Marc. *How We Age.* Philadelphia: Da Capro Press, 2011.

17. Brokaw, Sarah. *Fortytude.* New York: Hyperion Books, 2011.

18. Rosenblatt, Roger. *Rules for Aging: Resist Normal Impulses, Live Longer, Attain Perfection.* New York: Harcourt Inc., 2000.

19. Imber, Gerald. *Absolute Beauty: A Renowned Plastic Surgeon's Guide to Looking Young Forever.* New York: William Morrow, 2005.

20. Chittister, Joan. *The Gift of Years: Growing Older Gracefully.* New York: BlueBridge, 2008.

21. Perricone, Nicholas. *Ageless Face, Ageless Mind: Erase Wrinkles and Rejuvenate the Brain*. New York: Ballantine Books, 2007.

22. Kunin, Audrey. *The DermaDoctor Skinstruction Manual: The Smart Guide to Healthy Beautiful Skin and Looking Good at Any Age*. New York: Simon & Schuster, 2005.

23. Buettner, Dan. *The Blue Zones: Lessons for Living Longer from the People Who've Lived the Longest*. Washington, DC: National Geographic, 2008.

24. Freedman, Marc. *Prime Time: How Baby Boomers Will Revolutionize Retirement & Transform America*. New York: Public Affairs, 1999.

25. Braverman, Eric. *The Edge Effect: Achieve Total Health and Longevity with the Balanced Brain Advantage*. New York: Sterling Publishing Company, 2004.

26. Roizen, Michael. *RealAge: Are You as Young as You Can Be?* New York: HarperCollins Books, 1999.

27. Freedman, Marc. *The Big Shift: Navigating the New Stage Beyond Midlife*. New York: Public Affairs, 2011.

28. Deville, Nancy. *Healthy, Sexy, Happy: A Thrilling Journey to the Ultimate You.* Austin, Texas: Greenleaf Book Group Press, 2011.

29. Weil, Andrew. *Healthy Aging: A Lifelong Guide to Your Physical and Spiritual Well-Being.* New York: Alfred Knopf, 2005.

30. Cohen, Gene. *The Mature Mind: The Positive Power of the Aging Brain.* New York: Basic Books, 2005.

31. Plasker, Eric. *The 100 Year Lifestyle: Dr. Eric Plasker's Breakthrough Solution for Living Your Best Life, Every Day of Your Life.* Avon, Massachusetts: Adams Media, 2007.

32. Fossel, Michael, Greta Blackburn, and Dave Woynarowski. *The Immortality Edge: Realize the Secrets of Your Telomeres for a Longer, Healthier Life.* Hoboken, New Jersey: John Wiley & Sons, 2011.

33. Braverman, Eric. *Younger (Thinner) You Diet.* New York: Rodale Books, 2009.

34. Chang, Joseph. *The Aging Myth: Unlocking the Mysteries of Looking and Feeling Young.* North Fort Meyers, Florida: Aylesbury Publishing, 2011.

35. Rolls, Barbara, and Robert Barnett. *Volumetrics Weight-Control: Feel Full on Fewer Calories.* New York: HarperCollins Publishers, 2000.

36. Crowley, Chris, and Henry Lodge. *Younger Next Year: A Guide to Living Like 50 Until You're 80 & Beyond.* New York: Workman Publishing Co., 2004.

37. McKenna, David. *Retirement Is Not for Sissies: A Game Plan for Seniors.* Newberg, Oregon: Barclay Press, 2008.

38. Viorst, Judith. *Unexpectedly Eighty.* New York: Free Press, Simon & Schuster, 2010.

39. Marriott, Susannah. *1001 Ways to Stay Young Naturally.* New York: DK Publishing, 2007.

40. Warshofsky, Fred. *Stealing Time.* New York: TV Books, 1999.

41. Giampapa, Vincent, Ronald Pero, and Marcia Zimmerman. *The Anti-Aging Solution: 5 Simple Steps to Looking and Feeling Young.* Hoboken, New Jersey: John Wiley & Sons, 2004.

42. Small, Gary. *The Longevity Bible: 8 Essential Strategies for Keeping Your Mind Sharp and Your Body Young.* New York: Hyperion Books, 2006.

43. Wildman, Frank. *Change Your Age: Using Your Body and Brain to Feel Younger, Stronger, and More Fit.* Philadelphia: Da Capro Lifelong Press, 2010.

44. Kalb, John. *Winning at Aging.* Ashland, Oregon: Confluence Books, 2011.

45. Frank, Bill. *Bill Frank's Forever Young.* New York: HarperCollins Publishing, 2003.

46. Masley, Steven. *Ten Years Younger: The Amazing Ten-Week Plan to Look Better, Feel Better, and Turn Back the Clock.* New York: Broadway Books, 2005.

47. Somer, Elizabeth. *Age Proof Your Body: Your Complete Guide to Looking and Feeling Younger.* New York: McGraw Hill, 2006.

48. Beare, Sally. *50 Secrets of the World's Longest Living People.* Philadelphia: Da Capro Press, 2006.

49. Carstensen, Laura. *A Long Bright Future: An Action Plan for a Lifetime of Happiness, Health, and Financial Security*. New York: Broadway Books, 2009.

50. LaRoche, Loretta. *Juicy Living, Juicy Aging: Kick Up Your Heels – Before You're Too Short to Wear Them*. Carlsbad, California: Hay House, 2009.

51. Flanigan, Richard, and Kate Flanigan Sawyer. *Longevity Made Simple: How to Add 20 Good Years to Your Life: Lessons from Decades of Research*. Denver: Williams Clark Publishing, 2007.

52. Nuland, Sherwin. *The Art of Aging: A Doctor's Prescription for Well-Being*. New York: Random House, 2007.

53. Chopra, Deepak, and David Simon. *Grow Younger, Live Longer: 10 Steps to Reversing Aging*. New York: Harmony Books, 2001.

54. McKhann, Guy and Marilyn Albert. *Keep Your Brain Young: The Complete Guide to Physical and Emotional Health and Longevity*. New York: John Wiley & Sons, 2002.

55. Vaughan, Donald. *The Everything Anti-Aging Book: Discover the Secrets of Looking Young, Feeling Great, and Having Boundless Energy.* Avon, Massachusetts: Avon Media Corporation, 2002.

56. Reader's Digest. *Looking After Your Body: An Owner's Guide to Successful Aging.* Pleasantville, New York: Reader's Digest Association, 2001.

57. Bortz, Walter. *Living Longer for Dummies.* New York: Hungry Minds Inc., 2001.

58. Erickson, Mark et al. *Old Is the New Young.* Guilford, Connecticut: Globe Piquot Press, 2009.

59. Pratt, Steven. *SuperHealth: 6 Simple Steps, 6 Easy Weeks, 1 Longer, Healthier Life.* New York: Dutton, 2009.

60. Lindbergh, Reeve. *Forward From Here: Leaving Middle Age – and Other Unexpected Adventures.* New York: Simon & Schuster, 2008.

61. Mallek, Henry. *The New Longevity Diet: How to Stay Young, Stay Healthy, Stay Slim by Eating the Foods You Love.* New York: Putnam & Sons, 2001.

62. Adams, Charles. *The Complete Geezer Guidebook: Everything You Need to Know About Being Old and Grumpy.* Fresno, California: Quill Driver Books, 2006.

63. Altug, Ziya, and Tracy Gensler. *The Anti-Aging Fitness Prescription.* New York: Healthy Living Books, 2005.

64. Sutherland, Carolyn. *The Body Knows How to Stay Young: Healthy Aging Secrets from a Medical Intuitive.* Carlsbad, California: Hay House, Inc., 2008.

65. Bankson, Marjory Zoet. *Creative Aging: Rethinking Retirement and Non-Retirement in a Changing World.* Woodstock, Vermont: SkyLight Paths Publishing, 2010.

66. Seckel, Brooke Rutledge. *Save Your Face: The Revolutionary Non-Surgical 6-Step Facial Rejuvenation Program.* Concord, Massachusetts: Peach Publications, 2006.

67. Allen, K. Eileen. *I Like Being Old: A Guide to Making the Most of Aging.* Bloomington, Indiana: iUniverse, 2009.

68. Giampapa, Vincent, and Miryam Williamson. *Breaking the Aging Code: Maximizing Your DNA Function for Optimal Health*

and Longevity. North Bergen, New Jersey: Basic Health Publications, 2004.

69. Logan, Alan, Mark Rubin, and Phillip Levy. *Your Skin, Younger: New Science Secrets to Reverse the Effects of Age.* Naperville, Illinois: Cumberland House, 2010.

70. Mathieson, Sherrie. *Forever Cool: How to Achieve Ageless, Youthful, and Modern Personal Style for Women and Men.* New York: Clarkson Potter Publishers, 2006.

71. Perricone, Nicholas. *Forever Young: The Science of Nutrigenomics for Glowing, Wrinkle-Free Skin and Radiant Health at Every Age.* New York: 1st Atria Books, 2010.

72. Scott-Moncrieff, Christina. *Natural Health at 50: The Vital Guide to Living Longer and Looking Good.* Pleasantville, New York: Reader's Digest, 2001.

73. loe, Meika. *Aging Our Way: Lessons for Living from 85 and Beyond.* New York: Oxford University Press, 2011.

74. Henderson, Veronique, and Pat Henshaw. *Colour Me Younger.* London: Octopus Publishing Group, 2008.

75. Campbell, T. C., and T. M. Campbell. *The China Study.* Dallas, Texas: Ben Bella Books, 2005.

76. Nakhla, Tony. *The Skin Commandments: 10 Rules to Healthy, Beautiful Skin.* St. Louis, Missouri: Reedy Press, 2011.

77. Null, Gary. *Gary Null's Power Aging.* Waterville, Maine: Thorndike Press, 2003.

78. Cherniske, Stephen. *The Metabolic Plan: Stay Younger Longer.* New York: Ballantine Books, 2003.

79. Perls, Thomas, and Margery Hutter Silver. *Living to 100: Lessons in Living to Your Maximum Potential at Any Age.* New York: Basic Books, 1999.

80. Greenwood-Robinson, Maggie. *Wrinkle-Free: Your Guide to Youthful Skin at Any Age.* New York: Berkley Books, 2001.

81. Agin, Brent, and Sharon Perkins. *Healthy Aging for Dummies.* Detroit: Thorndike Press, 2009.

82. Jackson, Tracey. *Between a Rock and a Hot Place: Why fifty Is Not the NEW THIRTY.* New York: HarperCollins Publishers, 2011.

83. Samples, Pat. *Body Odyssey: Lessons from the Bones and Belly.* Minneapolis: Syren Book Co., 2005.

84. Goldberg, Elkhonon. *The Wisdom Paradox: How Your Mind Can Grow Stronger as Your Brain Grows Older.* New York: Gotham Books, Penguin Group, 2005.

85. Fonda, Jane. *Prime Time.* New York: Random House, 2011.

86. Vaillant, G. *Aging Well: Surprising Guideposts to a Happier Life.* Boston: Little, Brown and Company, 2002.

87. Sharma, Hari. *Freedom From Disease: How to Control Free Radicals, a Major Cause of Aging and Disease.* Fresno, California: Veda Publishing, 1993.

88. Oz, Mehmet. "Turn Up the Burn." *O, The Oprah Magazine* May 2012: 76–78.

89. Feuer, Ava. "The Latest Science on Aging." *O, The Oprah Magazine* May 2012: 136.

90. Singer, Thea. "Calming the Fat Away." *O, The Oprah Magazine* May 2012: 148.

91. Sellers, Ronnie, ed. *Fifty Things To Do When You Turn Fifty.* Portland, Maine: Ronnie Sellers Production, 2005.

92. Kirkwood, Tom. *Time of Our Lives.* New York: Oxford University Press, 1999.

93. Roizen, Michael, and Mehmet Oz. *You Being Beautiful: The Owner's Manual to Inner and Outer Beauty.* New York: Thorndike Press, 2009.

94. Chopra, Deepak, and Rudolph Tanzi. *Super Brain.* New York: Harmony Books, 2012.

95. Gupta, Sanjay. *Chasing Life.* New York: Wellness Central, 2008

96. Dychtwald, Ken and Joe Flower. *Age Wave.* New York: Bantam Books, 1990.

WEBSITE ARTICLES
TABLE OF AUTHORITIES

1. *Natural Products Insider.* Boomers Changing the Face of Aging. October 5, 2011. Web. http://www.naturalproductsinsider. com/news/2011/10/boomers-changing-the-face-of-aging.aspx

2. Darden, Kathryn. *Skin, Health and Beauty.* Skin care/anti-aging industry booming with baby boomers from $80 billion to $114 billion in 2015. September 22, 2011. Web. http://skin-healthbeauty.blogspot.com/search?q=anti-aging+industry

3. *BabyBoomers.com National Association of Baby Boomers.* Percentage of Baby Boomers Undergoing Plastic Surgery & Why You Should Know. February 24, 2012. Web. http:// www.babyboomers.com/percentage-of-baby-boomers-under-going-plastic-surgery-why-you-should-know/14250/

4. *WebMD. Healthy Beauty.* Reviewed by Laura Martin, MD. August 30, 2011. 19 Best Kept Hair Secrets. n.d. Web. http://www.webmd.com/beauty/hair-repair/ss/slideshow-best-kept-hair-secrets?ecd=wnl_day_090312&ctr=wnl-day-090312_ld-stry

5. Oz, Mehmet and Michael Roizen. Boost Metabolism with Spicy Foods for Weight Loss. *RealAge.com.* March 3, 2012. Web. http://www.realage.com/diet-weight-loss/boost-metabolism-spicy-foods-for-weight-loss

6. Smith, Jody. Baby Boomers and Inflammation: Saving Our Ancient Teeth. *EmpowerHER.* January 15, 2012. Web. http://www.empowher.com/dental-amp-oral-health/content/baby-boomers-and-inflammation-saving-our-ancient-teeth

7. *Clairsonic.com.* Clairsonic Sonic Cleansing Improves the Appearance of Mature Skin. *J. Am. Acad. Dermatol.* 2007. Web. http://demandware.edgesuite.net/aang_prd/on/demandware.static/Sites-Clarisonic-US-Site/Sites-Clarisonic-US-Library/default/v1391962119949/static_pages/clinical-studies/clarisonic-sonic-cleansing-improves-appearance-of-mature-skin.pdf

8. *FoodForTheBrain.org.* 6 Alzheimer's Prevention Steps. n.d. http://www.foodforthebrain.org/content.asp?id_Content=1821

9. *Healthy Aging.Net.* The Battle Cry for Aging: Vive La Change! July 9, 2009. Web. http://www.healthyaging.net/articlelive/articles/101/1/THE-BATTLE-CRY-FOR-AGING--VIVE--LA-CHANGE/Page1.html.

10. *RealAge.com.* Vitamin D Benefits: Clear Brain Plaques with This Nutrient. September 2011. Web. http://www.realage.com/health-tips/vitamin-d-prevents-alzheimers-plaques?eid=1010648261&memberid=12527912

11. Brunt, Mike. Question to Boomers...How Will You Live? *SeniorCare2Share.com.* January 18, 2011. Web. http://seniorcare-2share.com/2011/01/question-to-boomers-how-will-you-live

12. *US Department of Health and Human Services, National Institutes of Health.* Healthy Aging: Lessons from the Baltimore Longitudinal Study of Aging. Publication Date: July 2010. Last Updated: June 26, 2013. Web. http://www.nia.nih.gov/health/publication/healthy-aging-lessons-baltimore-longitudinal-study-aging/introduction.

13. *US Department of Health and Human Services, National Institutes of Health.* Healthy Aging: Can We Prevent Aging? July 2010. Web. http://www.nia.nih.gov/health/publication/

healthy-aging-lessons-baltimore-longitudinal-study-aging/
introduction. Last Updated: October 21, 2011.

14. Walters, Sheryl. Fresh Pineapple Has Many Benefits.
NaturalNews.com. February 28, 2009. Web. http://www.nat-
uralnews.com/025746_pineapple_fruit_Bromelain.html

15. Wilson, Tanya. Foods and Phytonutrients: Table of Potential
Benefits for Health and Weight Loss. *Dietivity.com.* November
22. Web. http://www.dietivity.com/foods-and-phytonutri-
ents-table-of-potential-benefits-for-health-and-weight-loss

16. Nichols, Joshua. 10 Simple Ways to Live Longer, Healthier.
ClickonDetroit.com. January 27, 2012. Updated September
14, 2012. Web. http://www.clickondetroit.com/lifestyle/
healthy-heart/10-simple-ways-to-live-longer-health-
ier/-/8499592/8510968/-/o9vvbnz/-/index.html

17. *NewsCore.* Teeth and Gums Reveal the Inside Story of
Your Overall Health. January 25, 2012.Web.http://www.
recordonline.com/apps/pbcs.dll/article?AID=/20120125/
HEALTH/201250302&emailAFriend=1

18. *WebMD. 25* Ways to Get Ready for Swimsuit Season. April 12, 2012. Web. http://www.webmd.com/diet/ss/slideshow-bikini-countdown?ecd=wnl_fit_040612

19. Oz, Mehmet and Michael Roizen. 5 Foods That Help You Sleep Better. *RealAge.* March 26, 2012. Web. http://www.realage.com/insomnia-and-sleep-problems/5-foods-that-help-you-sleep-better?eid=1010657189&memberid=13072830&cbr=SALE1200022

20. Oz, Mehmet and Michael Roizen. Can't Lose Weight? Try 7 Minutes of Meditation. *RealAge.* April 12, 2012. Web. http://www.realage.com/diet-weight-loss/do-meditation-to-lose-weight?eid=1010663375&memberid=13072830

21. *FoodfortheBrain.org* Food for the Brain E-News. "Healthy Body, Healthy Brain?" April 2012. Web. http://www.foodforthebrain.org/publications-and-events/e-news.aspx

22. *WebMD.* Slimming Slideshow: 24 Ways to Lose Weight Without Dieting. April 27, 2012. Web. http://www.webmd.com/diet/ss/slideshow-no-diet-weight-loss?ecd=wnl_day_042512

23. *WebMD*. Slideshow. 18 Secrets for a Longer Life. April 2012. Web. http://www.webmd.com/healthy-aging/ss/slideshow-longer-life-secrets?ecd=wnl_lbt_042512

24. *RealAge.com*. Double-Duty Exercise Opportunities. August 2009. Last reviewed June 1, 2009. Web. http://www.realage.com/fitness/double-duty-exercise-opportunities?src=edit&chan=tip&con=tip&click=p5

25. Templeton, Hollis. 10 Weird (and Wonderful) Weight Loss Side Effects. *Fitbie.com*. April 30, 2012. Web. http://fitbie.msn.com/slideshow/10-weird-and-wonderful-weight-loss-side-effects/slide/1

26. Oz, Mehmet and Michael Roizen. 8 Top Foods to Eat for Healthy Hair. *RealAge.com*. May 3–4, 2012. Web. http://www.realage.com/food/top-8-foods-for-healthy-hair?eid=1010657296&memberid=13072830

27. *WebMD*. *Healthy Beauty*. Top 10 Foods for Healthy Hair. Reviewed July 6, 2011. Web. http://www.webmd.com/healthy-beauty/features/top-10-foods-for-healthy-hair?page=3

28. *WebMD daily.* 24 Ways to Lose Without Dieting. Reviewed by Louise Chang. August 10, 2011. Web. http://www.webmd.com/diet/ss/slideshow-no-diet-weight-loss?ecd=wnl_day_042512

29. *Dentistry iQ News* (reported by American Academy of Periodontology "This Week in Perio"). Brushing your teeth could save your life. Copyright 2012. Web. http://www.dentistryiq.com/news/2012/09/13/brushing-your-teeth-could-save-your-life.html

30. Editor, Helping You Care (reported by American Academy of Periodontology "This Week in Perio"). Dental Health Key to Good Physical Health, Experts Say. *Helping YouCare.* September 24, 2012. Web. http://www.helpingyoucare.com/22391/dental-health-key-to-good-physical-health-experts-say

31. Sheriff, Natasja.Editing by Elaine Lies and Bob Tourtellotte. Dental Health Linked to Dementia Risk: Study (reported by American Academy of Periodontology "This Week in Perio"). *Reuters Health;* August 21, 2012. Web. http://www.reuters.com/article/2012/08/21/health-dementia-teeth-idUSL4E8JL00020120821

32. *Medicalxpress.* (reported by American Academy of Periodontology "This Week in Perio"). Oral bacteria may signal pancreatic cancer risk. *This Week in Perio.* Web. September 18, 2012. http://medicalxpress.com/news/2012-09-oral-bacteria-pancreatic-cancer.html

33. *WebMD.* Non-Surgical Cosmetic Procedures for the Face. Reviewed by Laura Martin, MD. December 16, 2011. Web. http://www.webmd.com/healthy-beauty/ss/slideshow-non-surgical-facial--procedures?ecd=wnl_day_072312&ctr=wnl_day_072312_ld-stry

34. *WebMD.* What Your Hair & Scalp Say About Your Health. Reviewed by Emmy M. Graber, MD on April 29, 2012. Web. http://www.webmd.com/skin-problems-and-treatments/ss/slideshow-hair-conditions?ecd=wnl-day-071912&ctr=wnl-day-071912_ld-stry

35. Barker, Joanne. What Does Your Smile Say About You? (reported by American Academy of Periodontology "This Week in Perio"). by Alfred Wyatt, DMD on May 11, 2012. Web. http://www.webmd.com/healthy-beauty/beautiful-smile-12/smile-personality?page=2

36. *WebMD.* Look-Younger Secrets That Work. Reviewed by Kathy Empen, MD on November 22, 2011. Web. http://www.webmd.com/healthy-beauty/ss/slideshow-look-younger-secrets?ecd=wnl_day_051712

37. Oz, Mehmet and Michael Roizen. 7 Foods for Healthy Eyes. *RealAge.* Web. Copyright 2012. http://www.realage.com/eye-health/food-for-eyes?src=nl&dom=realage&list=aw&link=text&ad=contact-lenses-awareness&eid=1010663316&memberid=13072830#fbIndex

38. Dr. Blaylock on *Newsmax health.* Vitamins C and E Protect Brain. Copyright 2012 Newsmax. Web. http://www.news-maxhealth.com/dr_blaylock/vitamins_C_E_brain_protec/2012/08/02/466202.html?s=al&promo_code=FA4F-1

39. Ostrow, Nicole. Eating More Berries May Delay Memory Decline, Research Shows. *Bloomberg.com.* April 25, 2012. Web. http://www.bloomberg.com/news/2012-04-26/eating-more-berries-may-delay-memory-decline-research-shows.html

40. Holford, Patrick. How to Stop Your Brain Aging. *Food for the Brain E-News.* Copyright 2012. Web.

41. O'Connor, Anahad. Really? Gum Disease Tied to Pancreatic Cancer Risk. Published in the *New York Times* (reported by American Academy of Periodontology "This Week in Perio"). October 1, 2012. http://well.blogs. nytimes.com/2012/10/01/really-gum-disease-tied-to-pancreatic-cancer-risk/

42. *WebMD*. Tips to Strengthen Your Immune System. Reviewed by Varanda Karriem-Norwood, MD. June 23, 2012. Web. http://www.webmd.com/diet/ss/slideshow-strengthen-immunity?ecd=wnl_day_080712&ctr=wnl-day-080712_ld-stry

43. Dr. Blaylock for *Newsmax.com*. Should I Take Vaccines? August 20, 2012. Web. http://www.newsmaxhealth. com/dr_blaylock/vaccine_risks/2012/08/20/469600. html?s=al&promo_code=FD81-1

44. Wanjek, Christopher. Want healthy knees? Focus on your gums. *Mother Nature Network*. June 26, 2012. Web. http://www.mnn.com/health/fitness-well-being/stories/ want-healthy-knees-focus-on-your-gums

45. Oz, Mehmet and Michael Roizen. How Flossing Is Linked to Overall Health. *RealAge*. March 8, 2012. Web. http://www.

realage.com/oral-care/how-flossing-is-linked-to-overall-healt
h?eid=1010657419&memberid=13072830

46. *FightAging.org.* A Discussion on Aging and the Immune System. November 10, 2010. Web. http://www.fightaging.org/archives/2010/11/a-discussion-on-aging-and-the-immune-system.php

47. Bouton, Katherine. Eighty Years Along, a Longevity Study Still Has Ground to Cover. *NY Times.* Books on Science book review. April 18, 2011. Web. http://www.nytimes.com/2011/04/19/science/19longevity.html?pagewanted=all&_r=0

48. Oz, Mehmet and Michael Roizen. Improve Memory with These Brain Boosters. *RealAge.* Published October 3, 2010. Web. http://www.realage.com/better-memory/improve-memory-brain-boosters?eid=1010677136&memberid=13072830

49. *WebMD.* Top Tips for Healthier Eyes. WebMD slideshow. Reviewed by Robert Butterwick, OD. May 7, 2013. Web. http://www.webmd.com/eye-health/ss/slideshow-healthier-eyes?ecd=wnl_day_021813&ctr=wnl-day-021813_ldstry&mb=

50. Grens, Kerry. Feeling stressed out tied to heart disease risk. *Heart Health, NBCNews.com.* September 27, 2012. Web. http://www.coreperformance.com/daily/live-better/high-stress-its-like-smoking-five-cigarettes-per-day-says-researcher.html

51. H*eraldonline.com* Gum disease treatment can lower annual medical costs for people with heart disease and stroke. February 26, 2013. Web. http://www.heraldonline.com/2013/02/26/4647891/gum-disease-treatment-can-lower.html

52. *WebMD.* Weight Loss Dos and Don'ts. Reviewed by Brunilda Nazario, MD. June 28, 2012. Web. http://www.webmd.com/diet/rm-quiz-weight-loss-dos-and-donts?ecd=wnl_wlw_031613&ctr=wnl-wlw-031613_ld-stry&mb=

53. *Newswise.* Literature Review Shows Inflammation Links Obesity and Gum Disease. Released March 11, 2013. Web. http://www.newswise.com/articles/literature-review-shows-inflammation-links-obesity-and-gum-disease

54. Zeisel, John. Want to age well? Learn New Tricks, Not Facts. *Nextavenue, org.* March 1, 2013. Web. http://www.nextavenue.org/article/2013-02/want-age-well-learn-new-tricks-not-facts

55. *WebMD*. 5 Foods for Better Vision. Posted May 16, 2013. Huff Post Post50. Web. http://www.huffingtonpost.com/2013/05/16/foods-for-vision_n_3280781.html?utm_hp_ref=fifty&ir=Fifty

56. *You Tube*. Video: ABC Prime Time Report on Protandim with John Quinones. Uploaded May 4, 2008. Web. http://www.abcliveit.com/site/ABC_Primetime_Report.html

57. Rosen, Margery. 7 Delicious Steps to a Stronger Memory. *AARP*. *Ju*ne 24, 2013. Web. http://www.aarp.org/health/brain-health/info-06-2013/worried-about-your-memory.5.html.

58. *HealthLink on King 5.com*. Skipping breakfast could increase heart attack risk. Posted June 22, 2013. Web. http://www.king5.com/health/Skipping-breakfast--216495181.html

59. Nierenberg, Carl. Pancreatic Cancer: Bacteria May Play a Role. (reported by the American Academy of Periodontology This Week in Perio"). July 23, 2103. Web. https://blu169.mail.live.com/default.aspx#n=1521234984&fid=d920087768c4cb39ea3dce070bd5c9c&mid=418e5890-f9d8-11e2-a5c5-00237de4b074

60. *WebMD*. Reviewed by Kathleen Zelman. Fat-Fighting Foods. October 4, 2011. Web. http://www.webmd.com/diet/ss/slide-show-fat-fighting-foods?ecd=wnl_day_082813&ctr=wnl-day-082813_ld-stry&mb=

61. Kingson, George. *CDAPress.com* (reported by the American Academy of Periodontology This Week in Perio"). Gum disease could lead to other problems. September 8, 2013. Web. http://www.cdapress.com/news/local_news/article_38e2890d-c01e-5f29-a164-97e873943474.html

62. Sporre, Kathy. *Refined by Age*. 7 Affirmations for Positive Aging. September 23, 2013. Blog. http://refinedbyage.com/2013/09/23/7-affirmations-for-positive-aging/

63. Gupta, Sanjay. In answer to Twitter question: What are Phytonutrients and why do we need them? *CNNhealth.com*. July 24, 2009. Web. http://thechart.blogs.cnn.com/2009/07/24/what-are-phytonutrients-and-why-do-we-need-them/

64. *National Institute on Aging*. Disability among older Americans continues significant decline. December 1, 2006. Web http://www.nia.nih.gov/newsroom/2006/12/disability-among-older-americans-continues-significant-decline

Made in the USA
Charleston, SC
01 October 2014